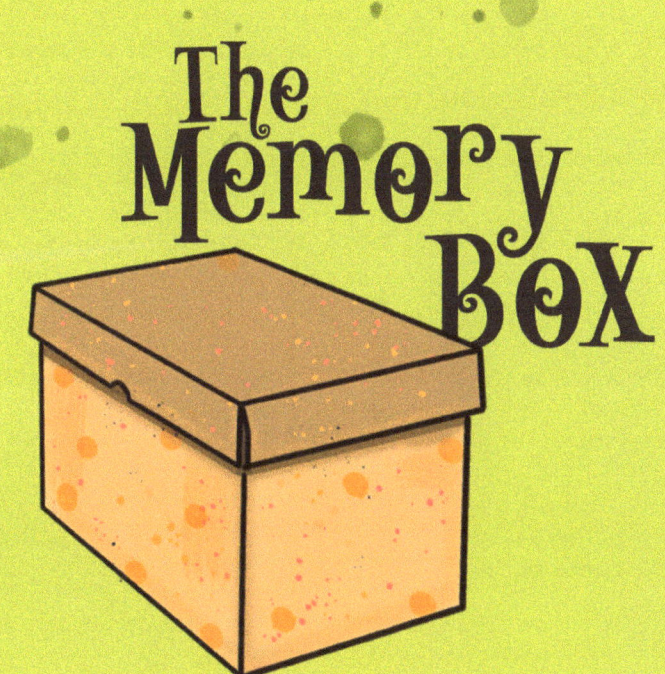
The Memory Box

The Memory Box & Charlotte's Big Surprise

Library of Congress Control Number: 2024915763

ISBN: 979-8-9888044-5-1 Hardback | ISBN: 979-8-9888044-7-5 Paperback

© 2025 by The Hartage Foundation Inc. All rights reserved. No part of this book may be reproduced or transmitted in any form or by any means, electronic or mechanical, including photocopy, recording, or any storage and retrieval system now or to be invented without written permission from the publisher. Contact: The Hartage Foundation, Inc. 1405 South Orange Ave. Suite 324, Orlando, Florida 32806. The layout, illustrations, drawings, and artwork are trademarks of the Hartage Foundation, Inc. and the author, Homer L. Hartage.

This book may be ordered directly from the author, but please try your local bookstore first. You may visit us at www.agedcareguardian.com or call us at 321-221-4351 or email: homer.hartage@agedcareguardian.com.

Other books by the author: Family and Professional Guardianship, ISBN: 979-8-98880443-0-6 Hardback, ISBN: 979-8-9888044-1-3 Paperback, ISBN: 979-8-9888044-2-0 Kindle, ISBN: 979-8-9888044 4-4 eBook.

Publisher: IngramSpark for The Hartage Foundation, Orlando, Florida USA

Written by: Homer L. Hartage
Creative Direction and Illustrations: Zohra Lakhani
Character Illustrations: Trúc Đăng
Editor: E. Lee Caleca
Cover design formatting: The Book Cover Whisperer

To my beloved Uncle Jonah
— A man of boundless energy, unwavering faith, and deep devotion to family. A proud Marine, a guiding role model, a joyful presence, and a Deacon whose spirit lifted everyone around him. Your love of life and the enduring memories you give inspire us.

              We will always remember you.

For the cherished memories of my brother Alonzo
— A radiant soul with a larger-than-life presence, whose laughter filled every room and whose heart embraced everyone he met. Your spirit continues to inspire and uplift us.

                   Love ya, man.

INTRODUCTION

When Charlotte's beloved Grandpa no longer recognizes her face or remembers her cherished name, her world crumbles in confusion. Desperate to reclaim their unbreakable bond, Charlotte embarks on a race against time to reawaken the memories that have slipped away from her grandpa.

Armed with a Memory Box filled with photographs and treasured moments, Charlotte embarks on an emotional journey of rediscovery, fueled by the hope that her grandpa will remember her again. As Charlotte shares stories and sings their favorite song, a flicker of recognition sparks in her grandpa's eyes, leading to a heartwarming and triumphant ending that celebrates the enduring power of love and the resilience of the human spirit.

Told through the eyes of a child, this heartwarming tale explores the complexities of family ties and the profound impact of memory on our lives.

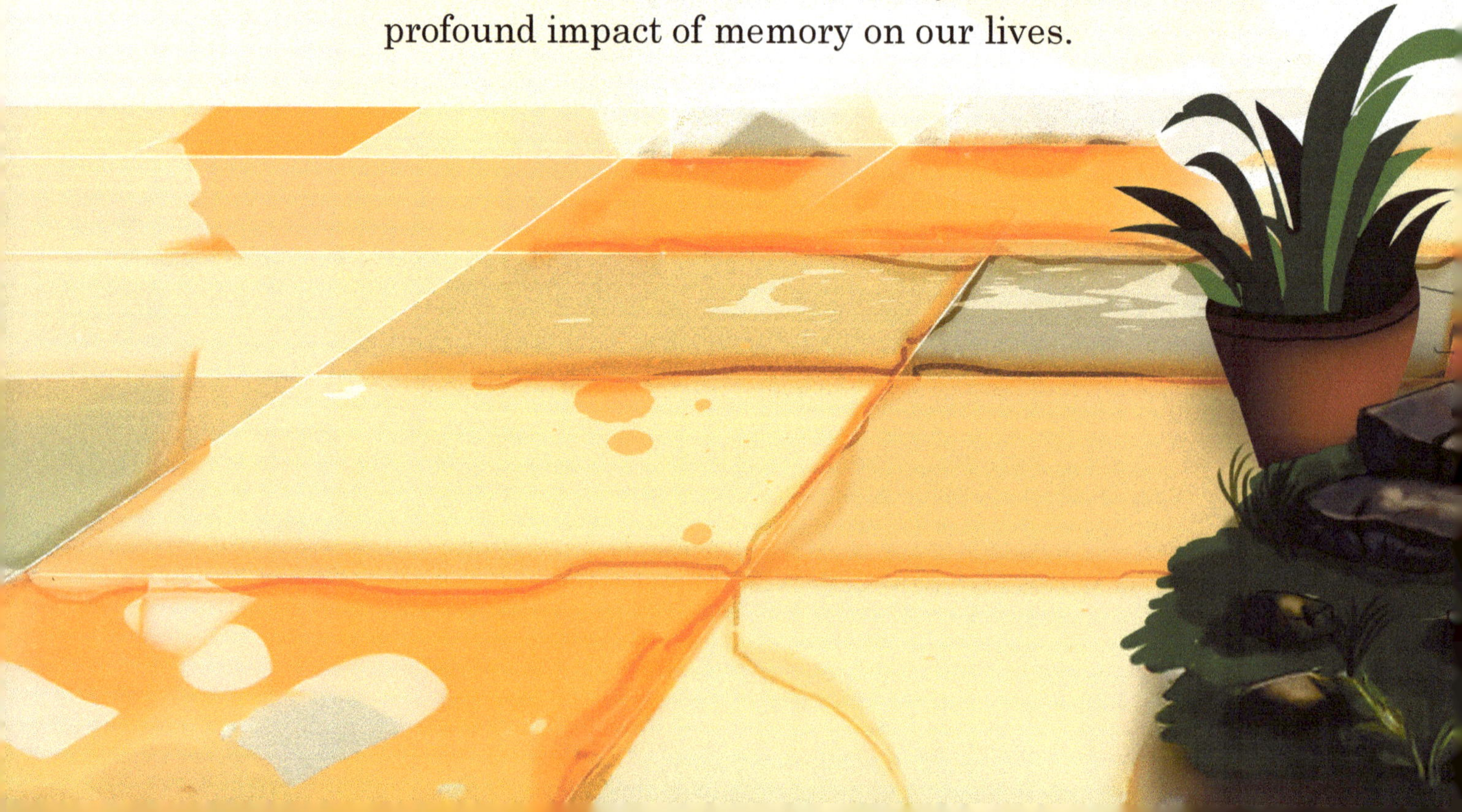

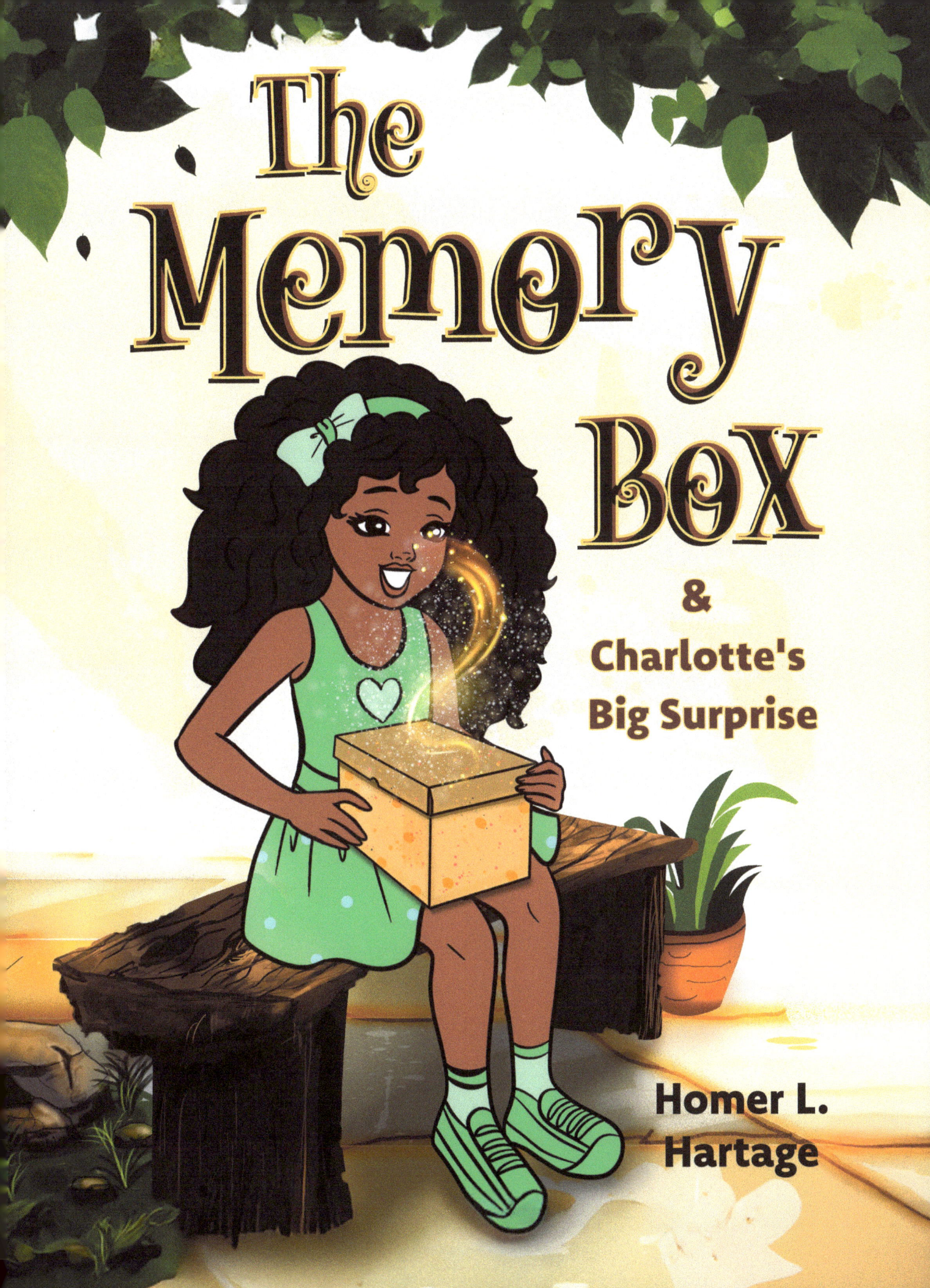

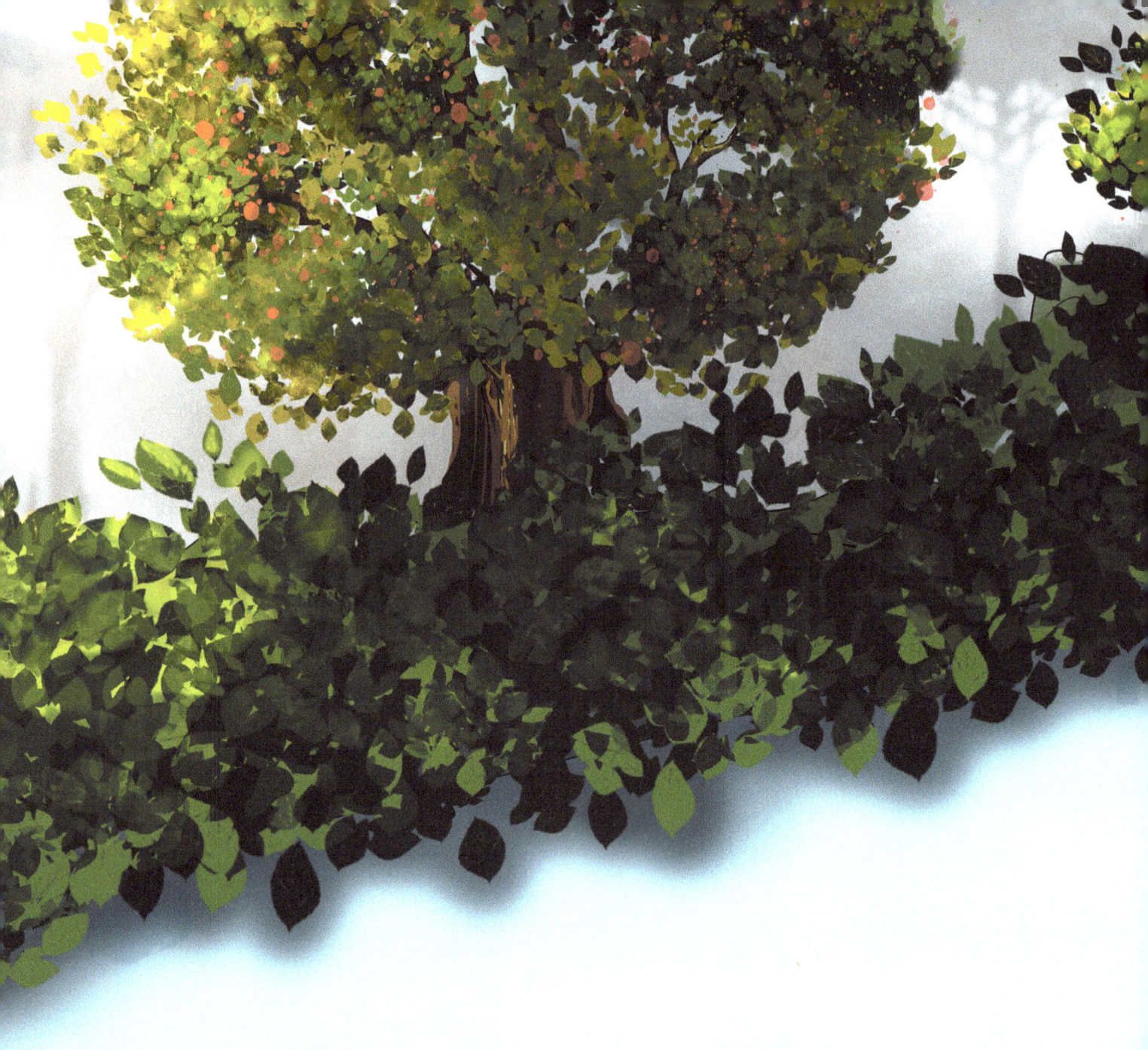

What was the big surprise?

Mom had been hinting for three days now about a big surprise.

What could it be?

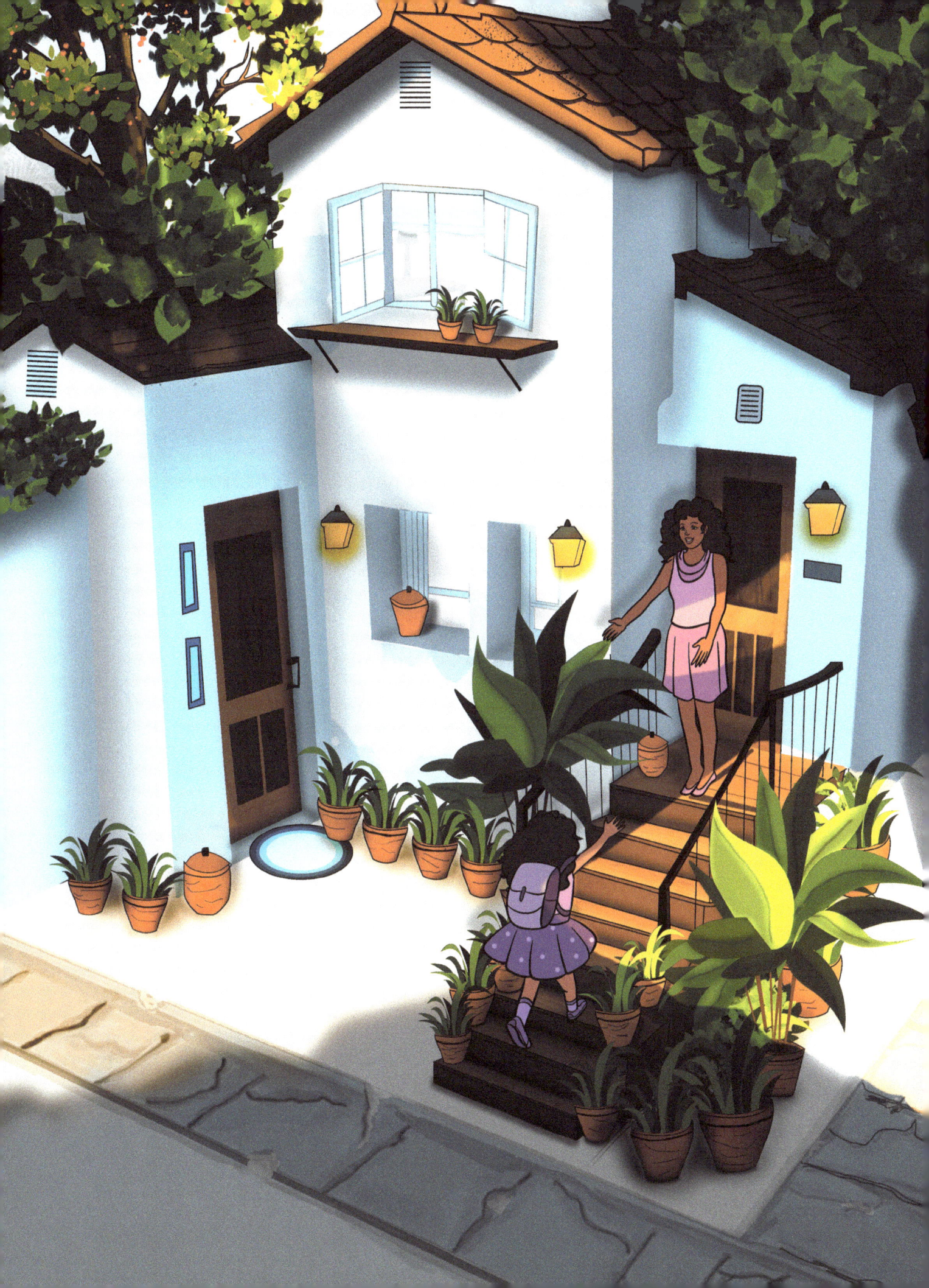

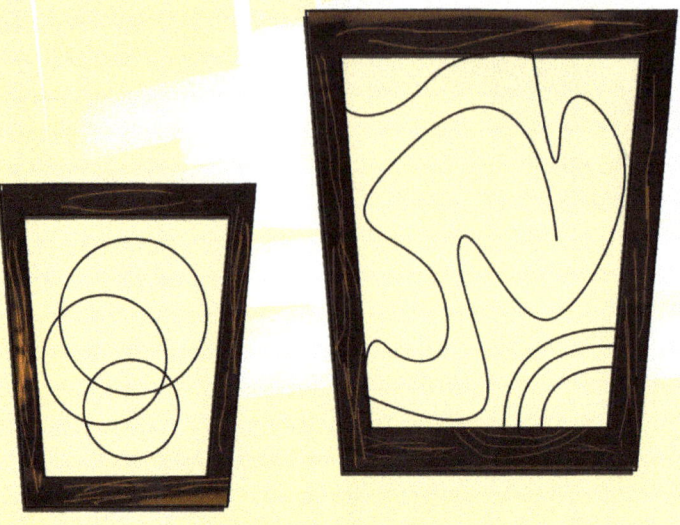

It was Friday, and I rushed home from school.
Again and again, I pleaded with her.
"What is the surprise?"

Mom just smiled, with a funny twist to her mouth.
"I will tell you today when your dad
gets home from work."

I sighed, crossing my arms over my chest.

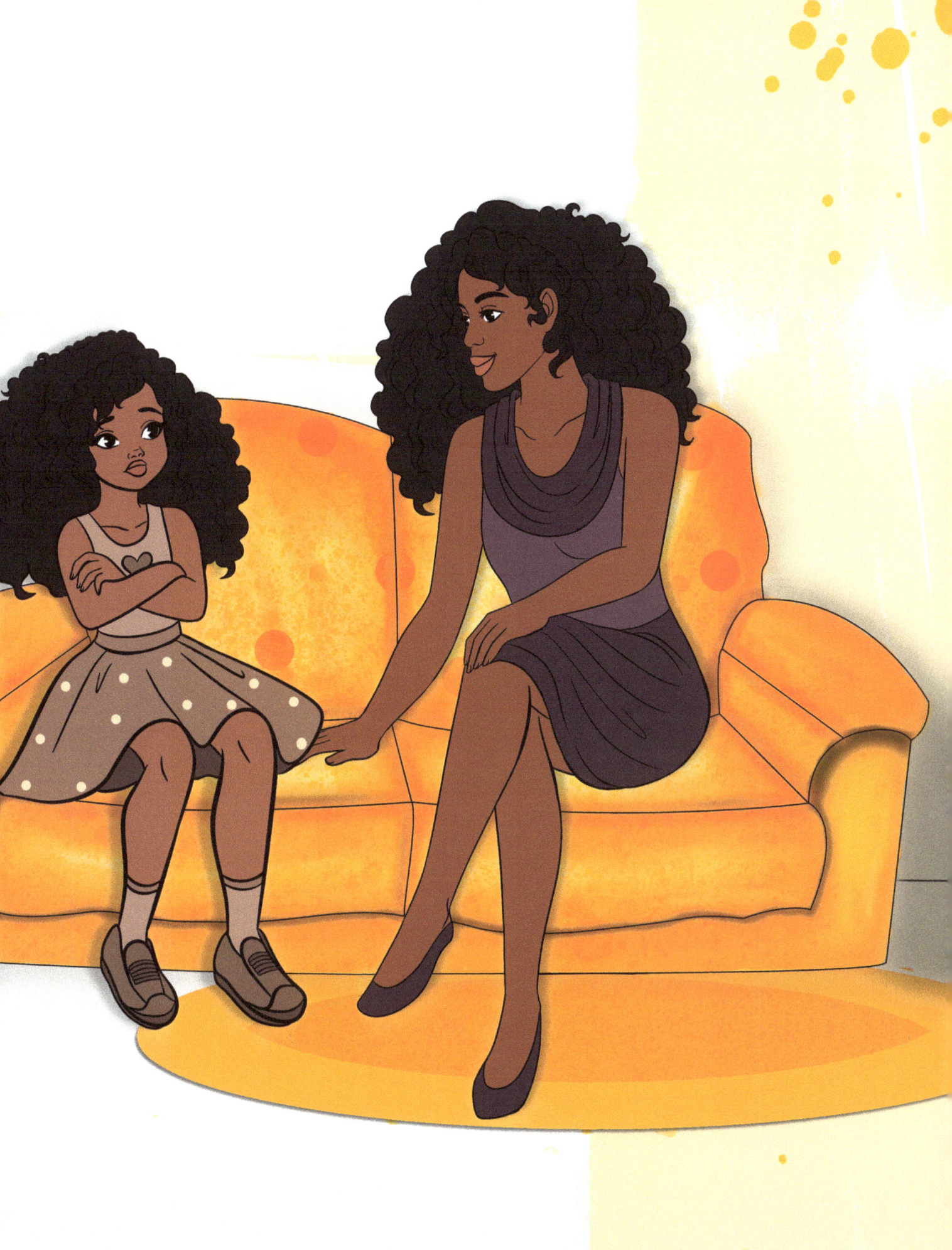

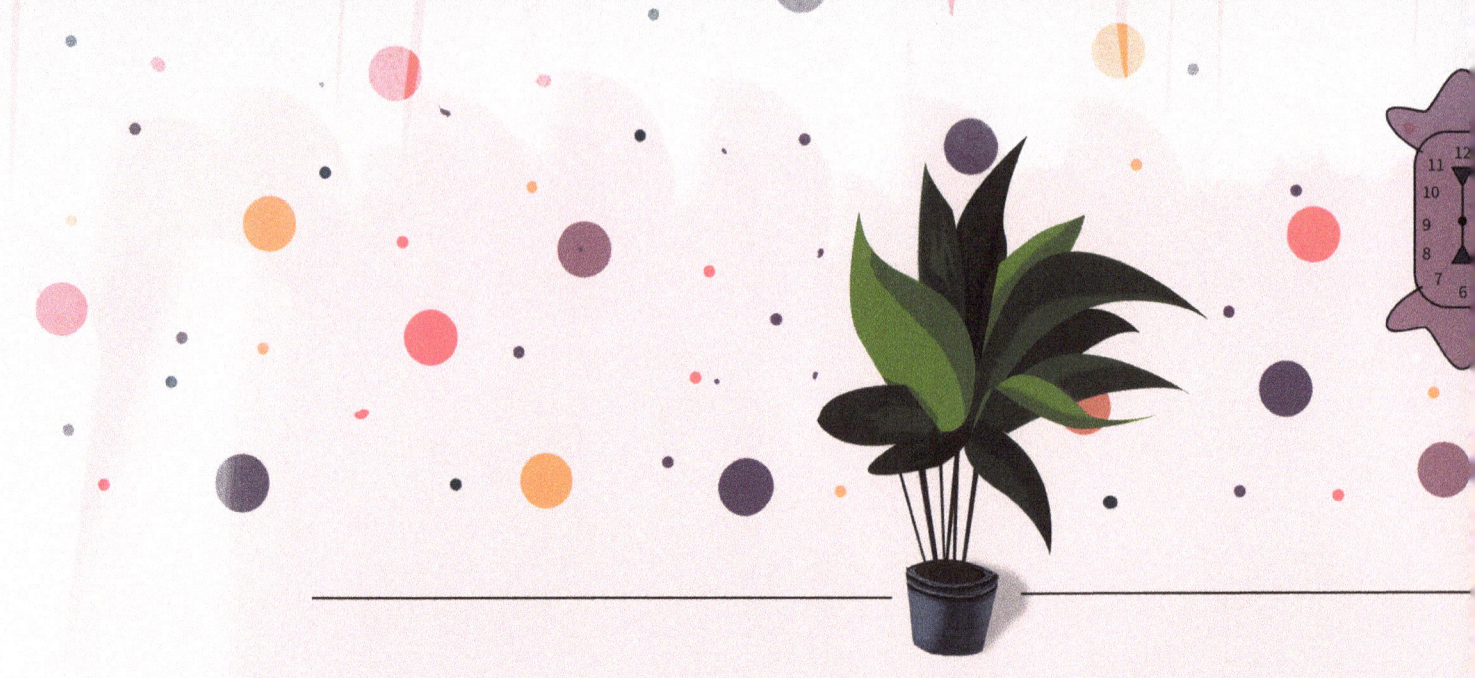

I watched the clock, waiting for it to turn to 6:00.
When Dad finally burst through the door,
he didn't give a hint of anything special.

He kissed Mom, and then
he picked me up and spun me around.

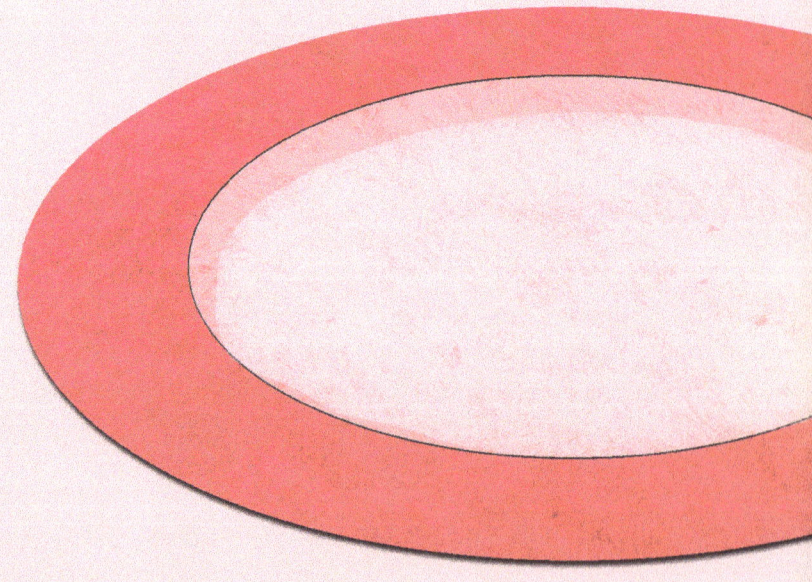

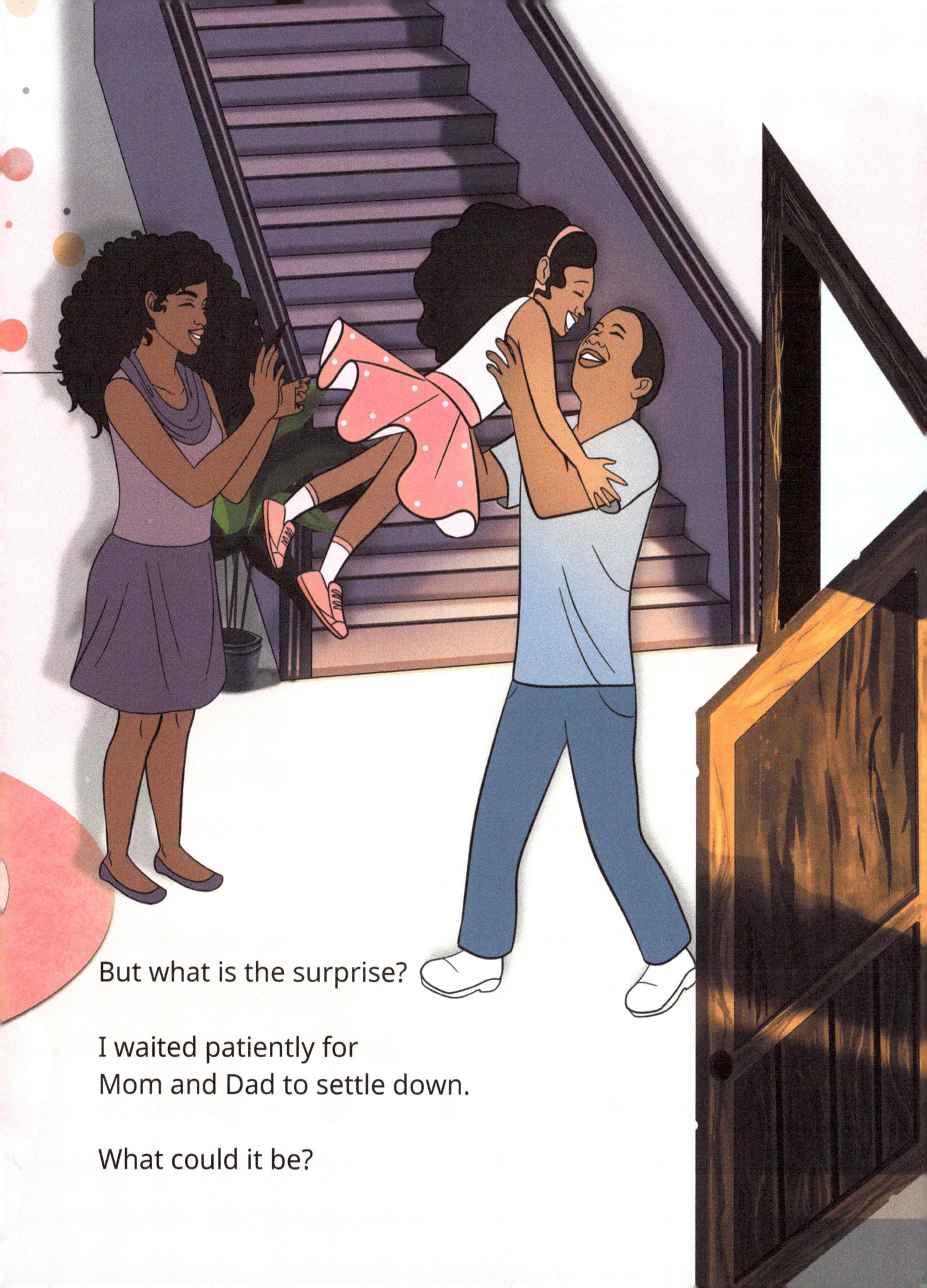

But what is the surprise?

I waited patiently for
Mom and Dad to settle down.

What could it be?

Mom could not hold it any longer. With a huge grin on her face, she kneeled and grabbed me by the shoulders.

"We are going to see Grandpa!"

I jumped and twirled around. "Grampa! Grampa! Grampa!"

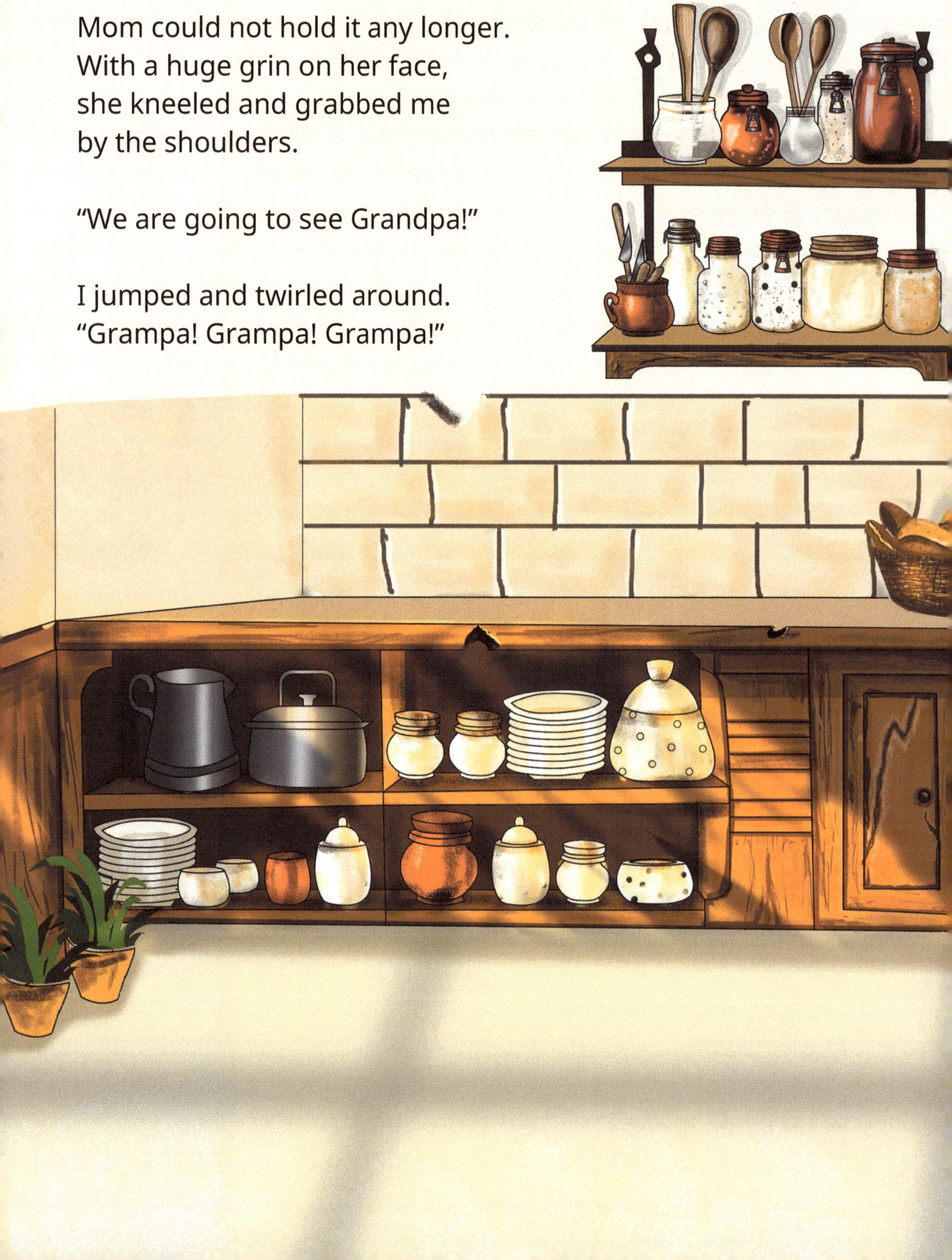

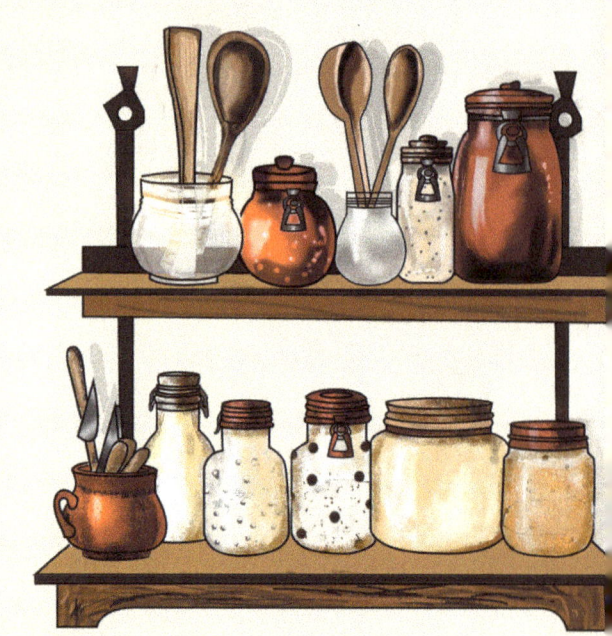

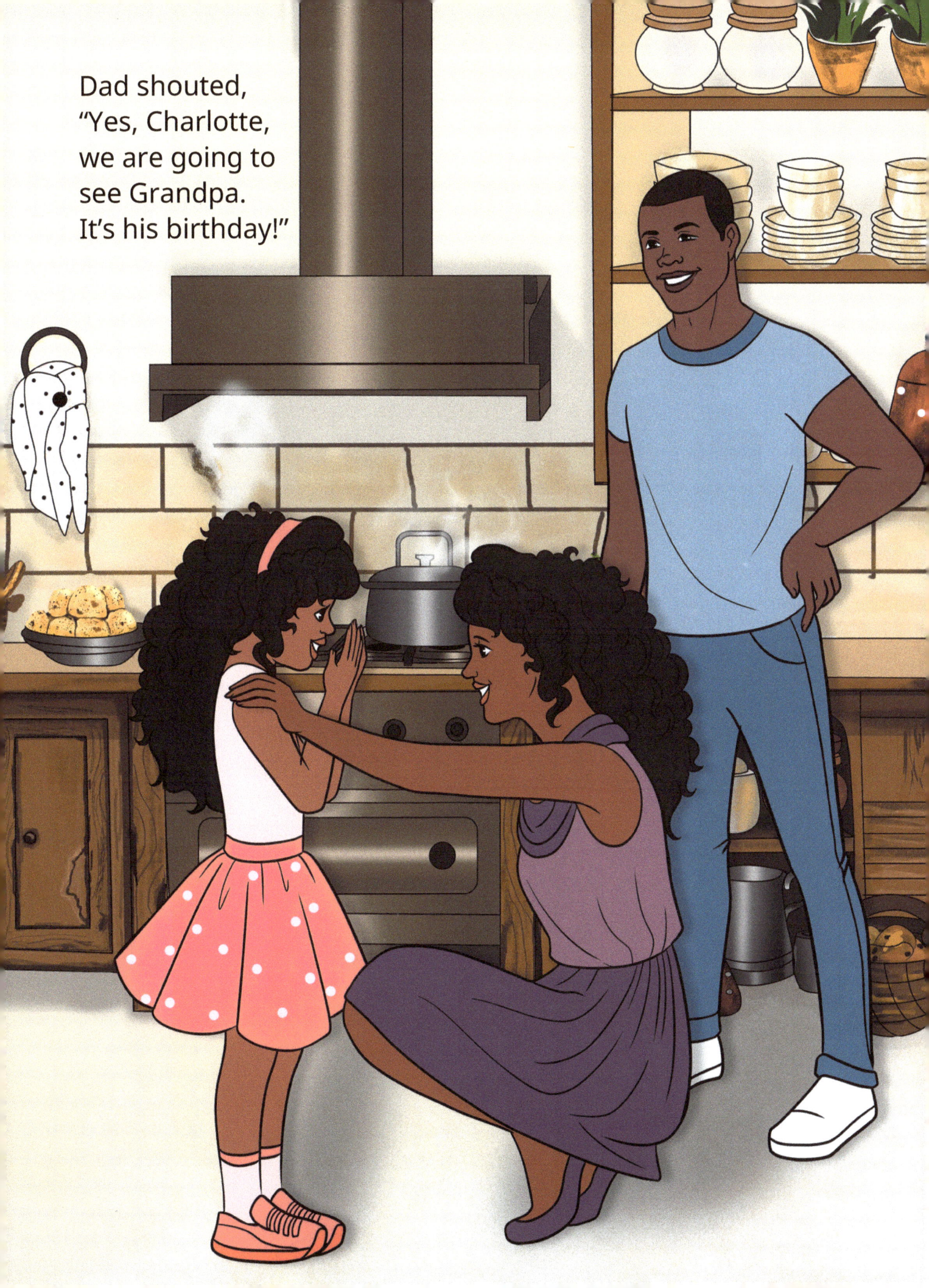

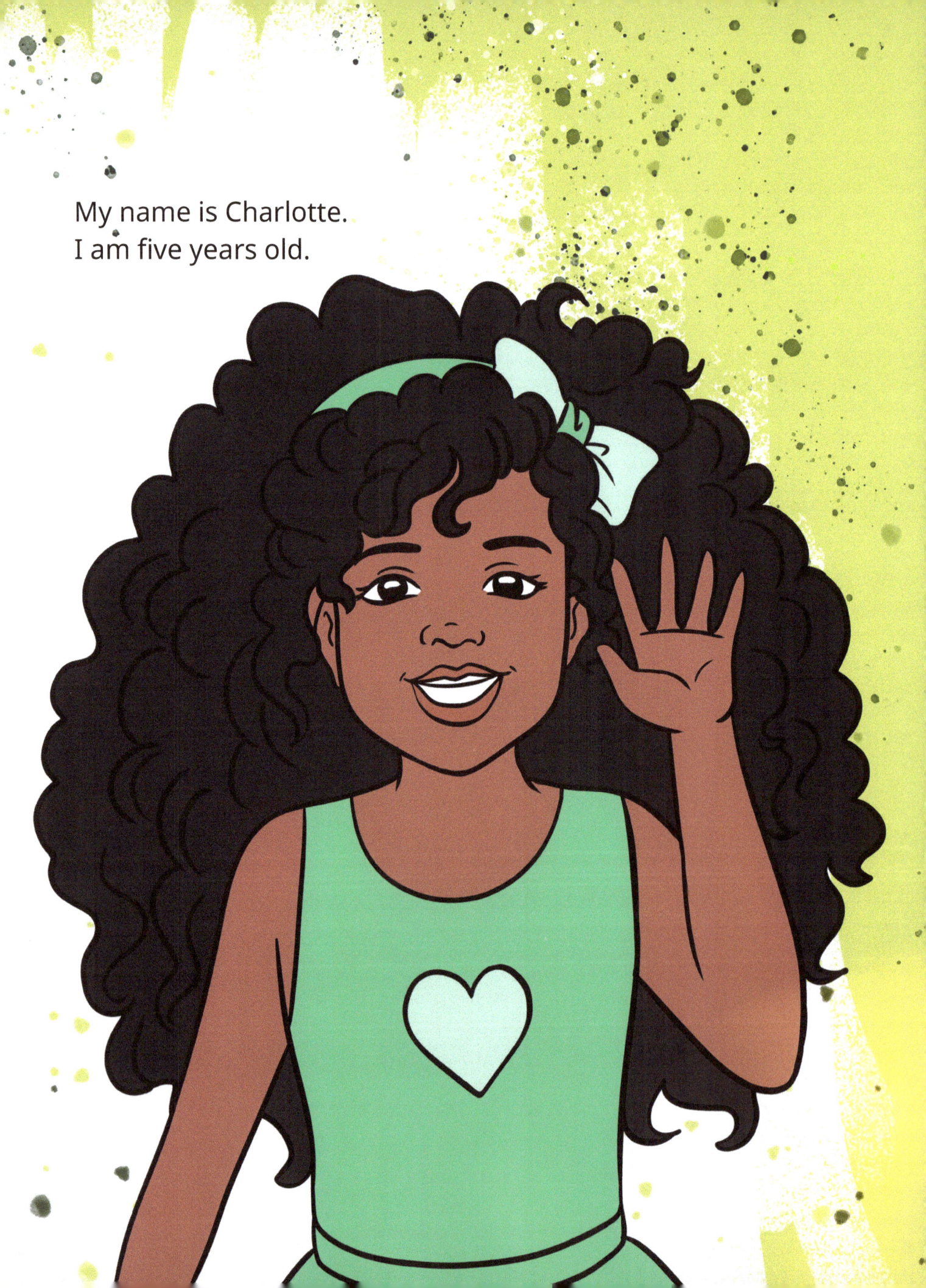

My name is Charlotte.
I am five years old.

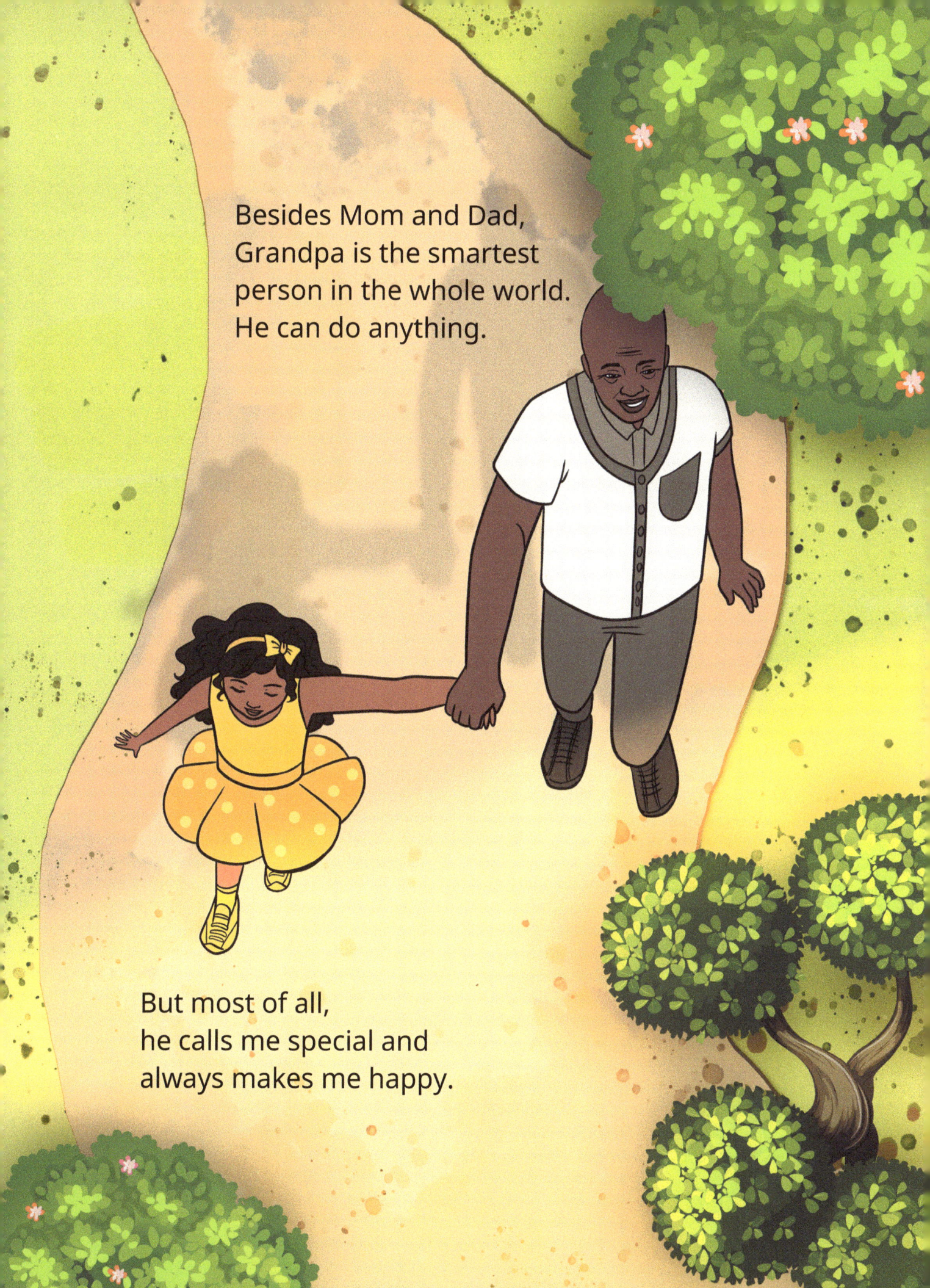

Besides Mom and Dad, Grandpa is the smartest person in the whole world. He can do anything.

But most of all,
he calls me special and always makes me happy.

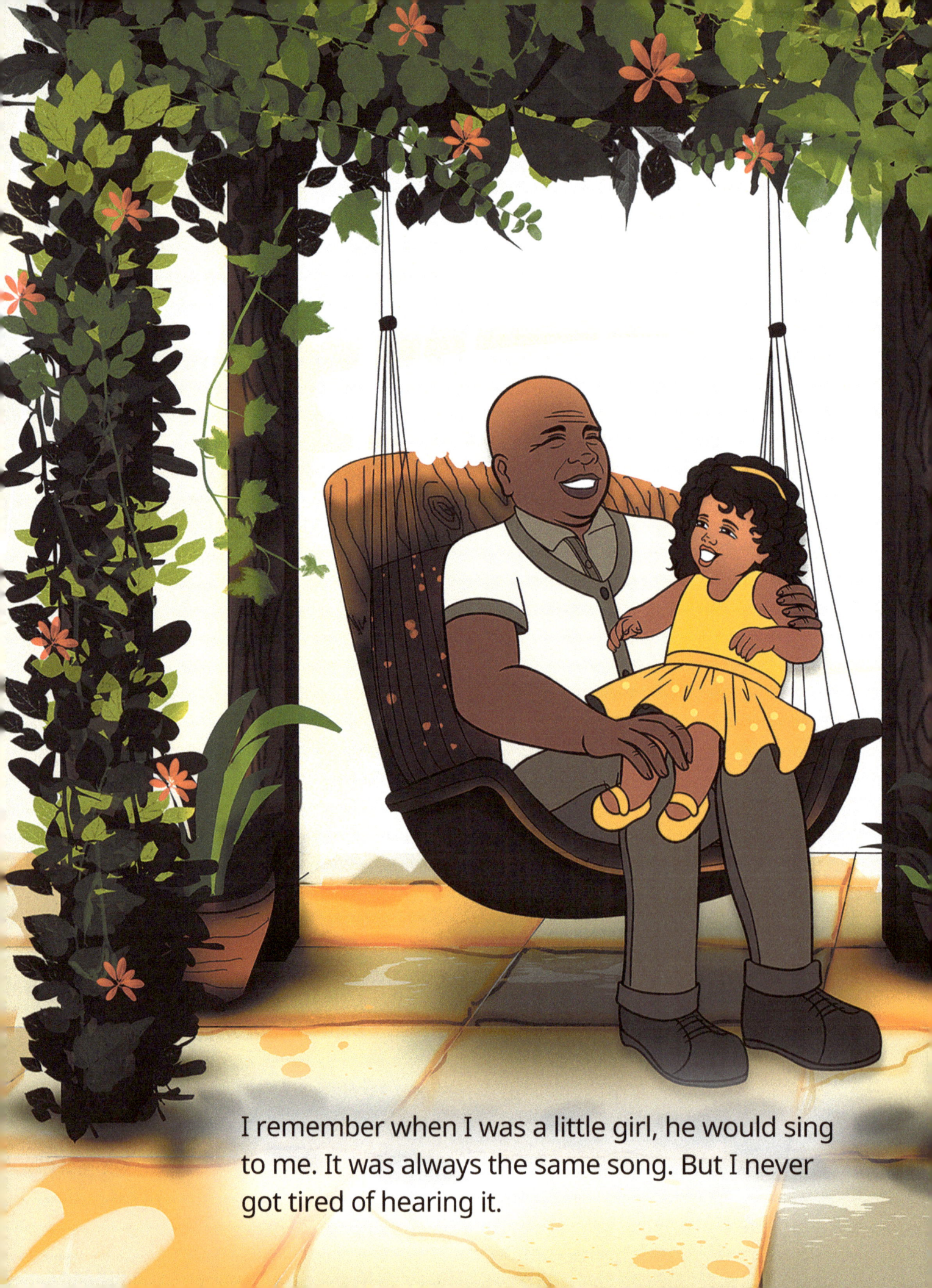

I remember when I was a little girl, he would sing to me. It was always the same song. But I never got tired of hearing it.

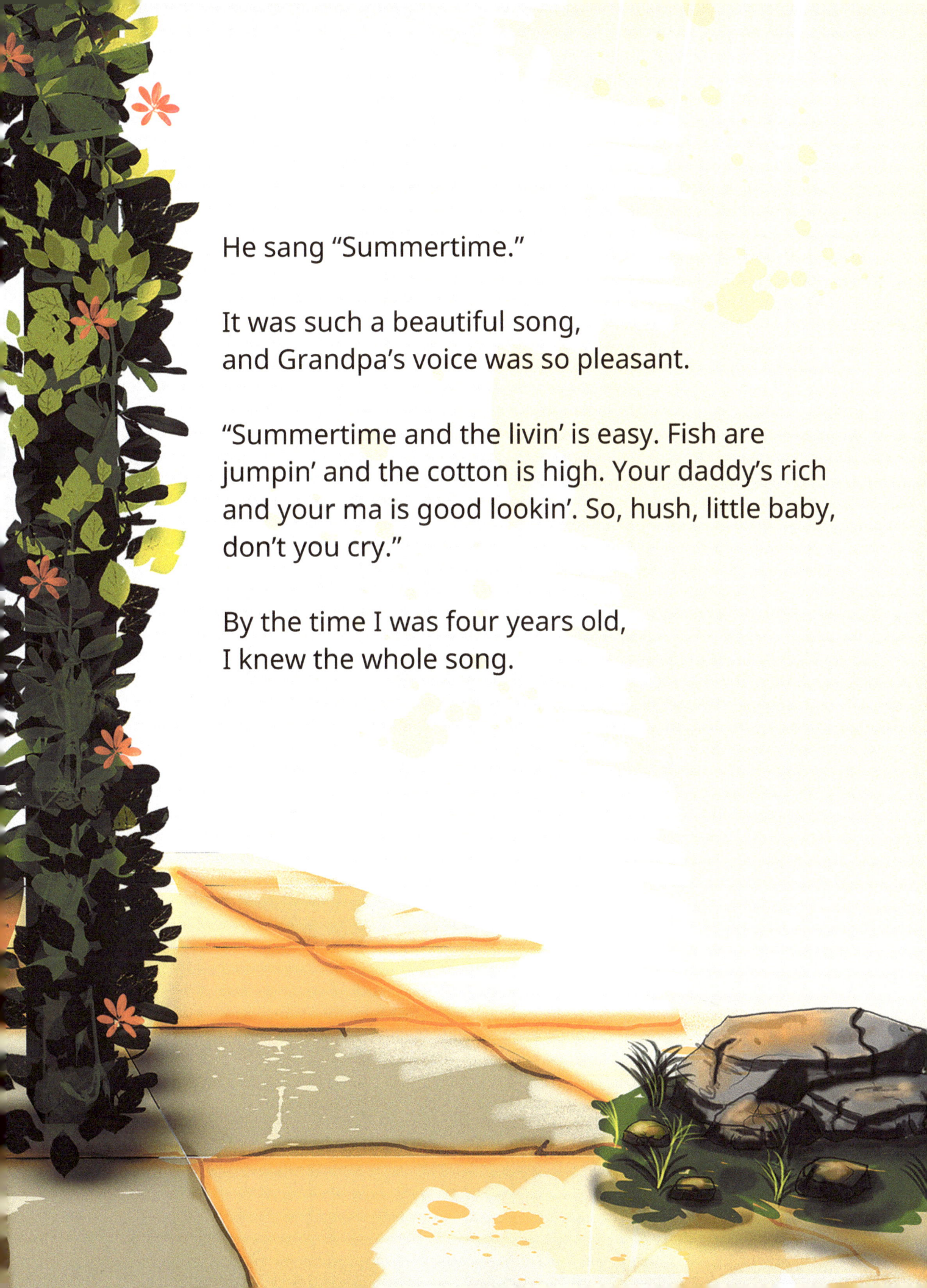

He sang "Summertime."

It was such a beautiful song,
and Grandpa's voice was so pleasant.

"Summertime and the livin' is easy. Fish are jumpin' and the cotton is high. Your daddy's rich and your ma is good lookin'. So, hush, little baby, don't you cry."

By the time I was four years old,
I knew the whole song.

Everyone would say that I was precocious.
Well, I wasn't sure what that meant.

I knew I was good at a lot of things,
like science and math.
I guess you'd say I was smart, for a little kid.

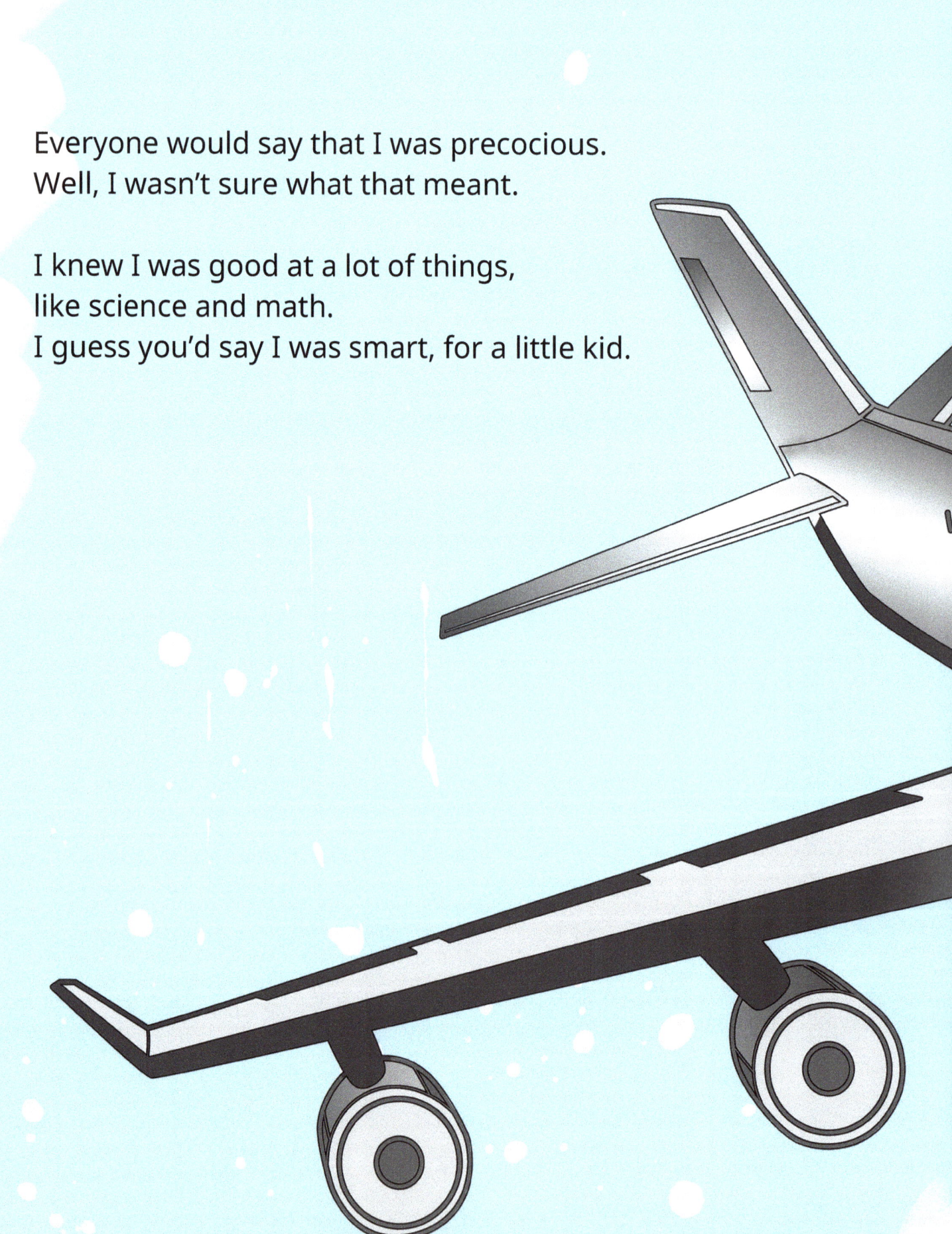

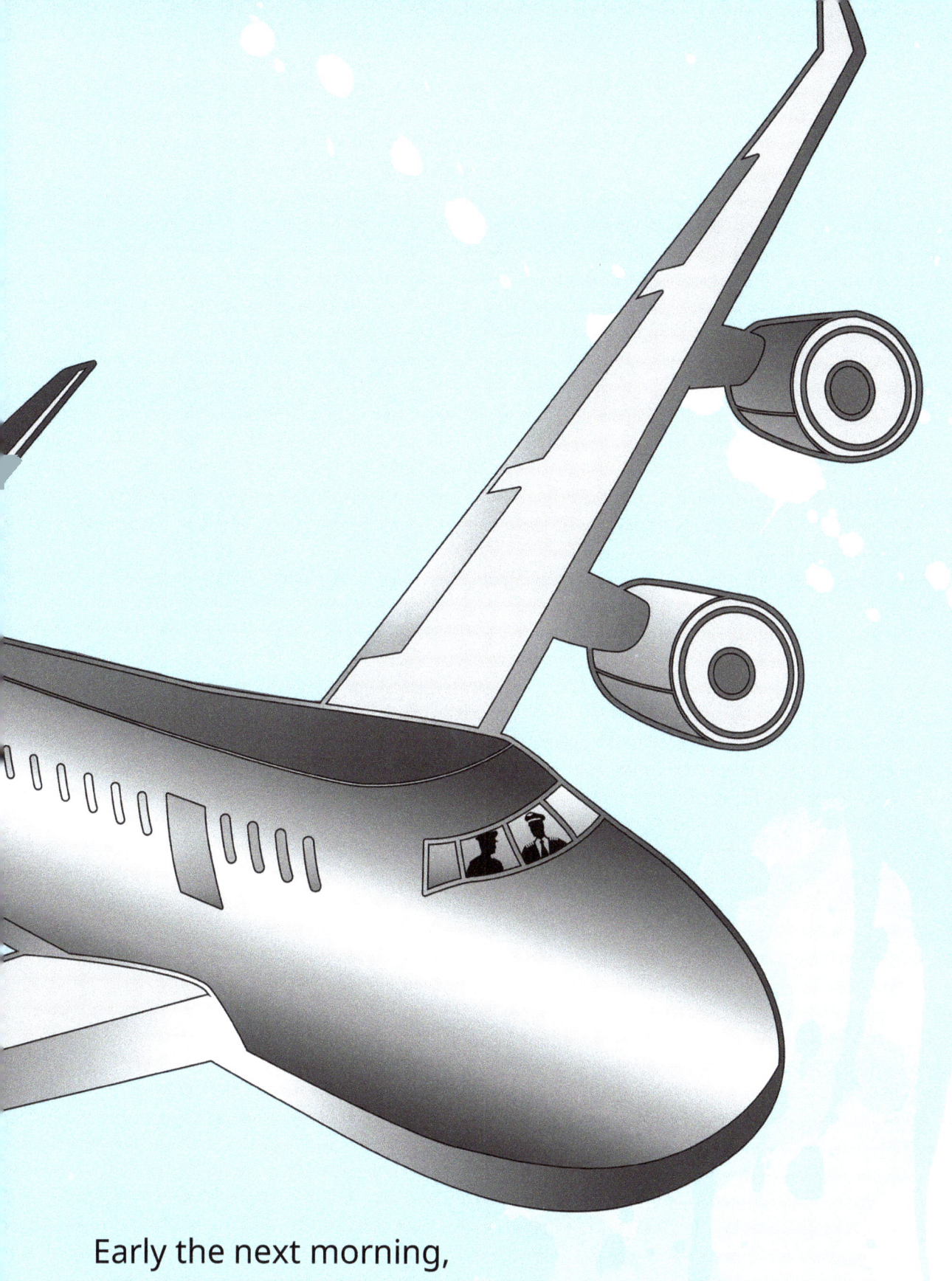

Early the next morning, we boarded a big, silver airplane.

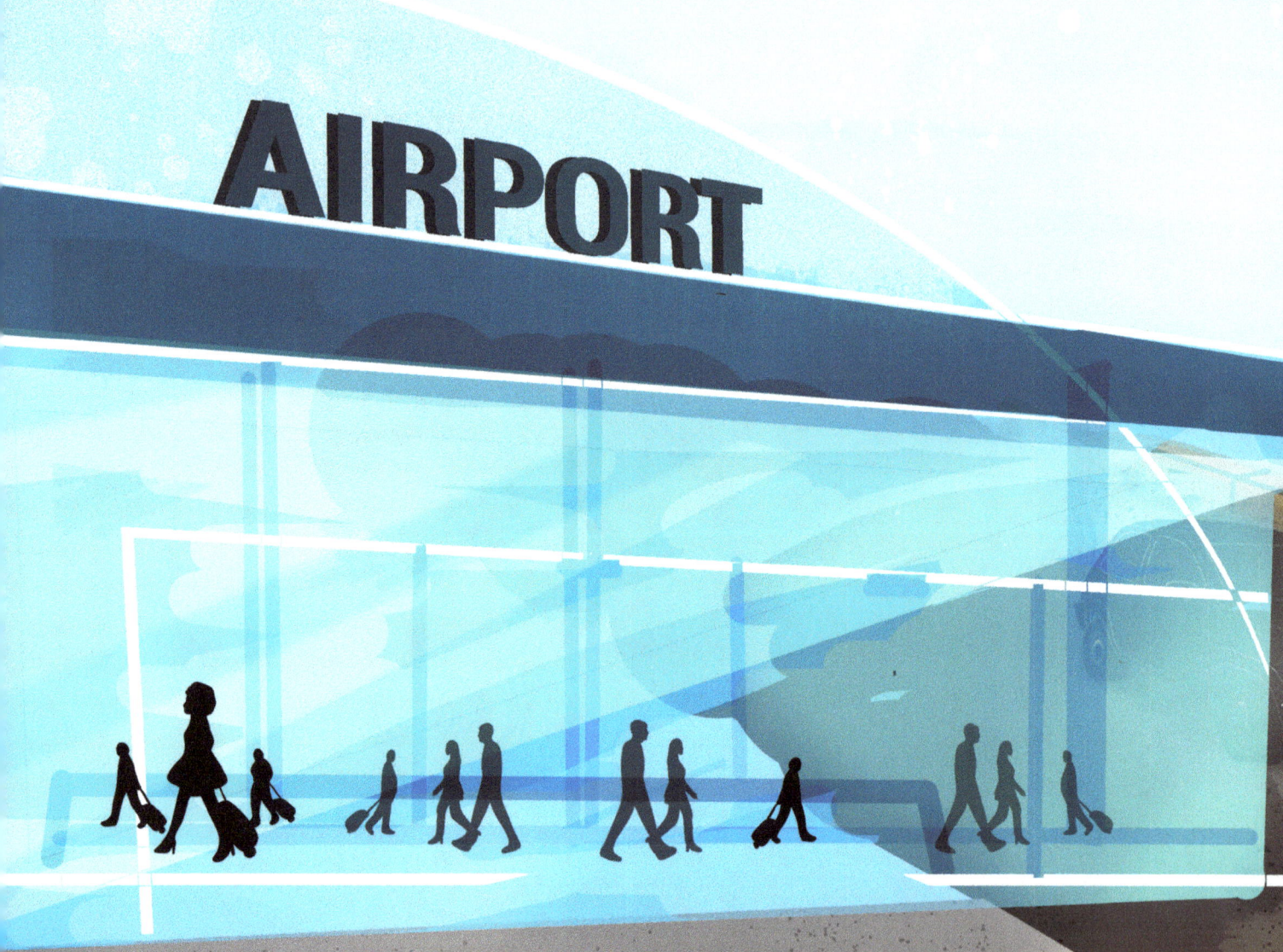

We arrived in Florida at noon.

Grandma met us at the airport. *Where was Grandpa?* I wondered, then I said it out loud.

"Where is Grandpa?"

"You will see him soon," Dad said, as we walked toward Grandma's car.

Grandma pressed a button, and the trunk opened. Dad loaded our bags into the car.

This car was really big to me. It had four doors and was blue, like the lake we went to last summer.

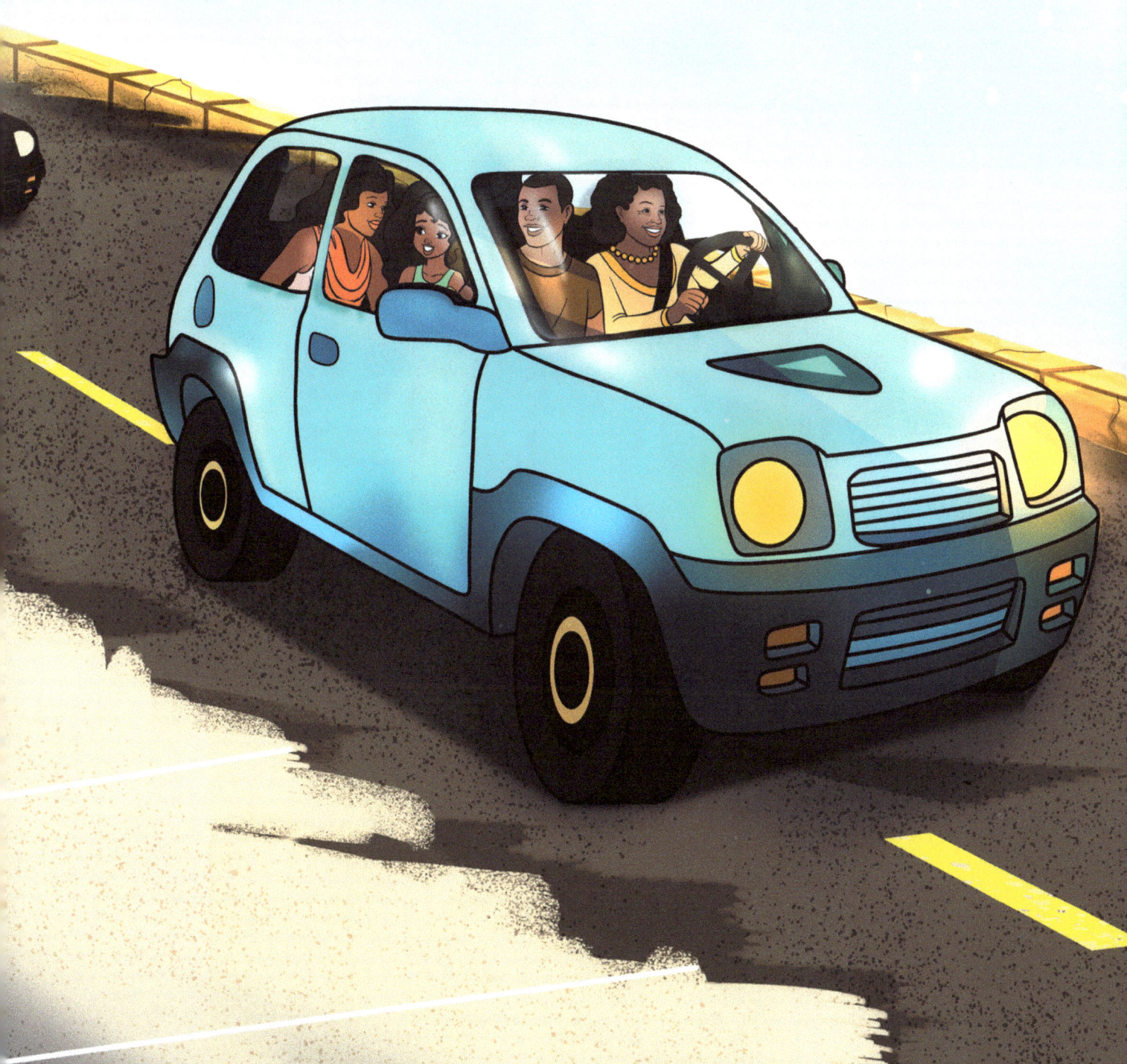

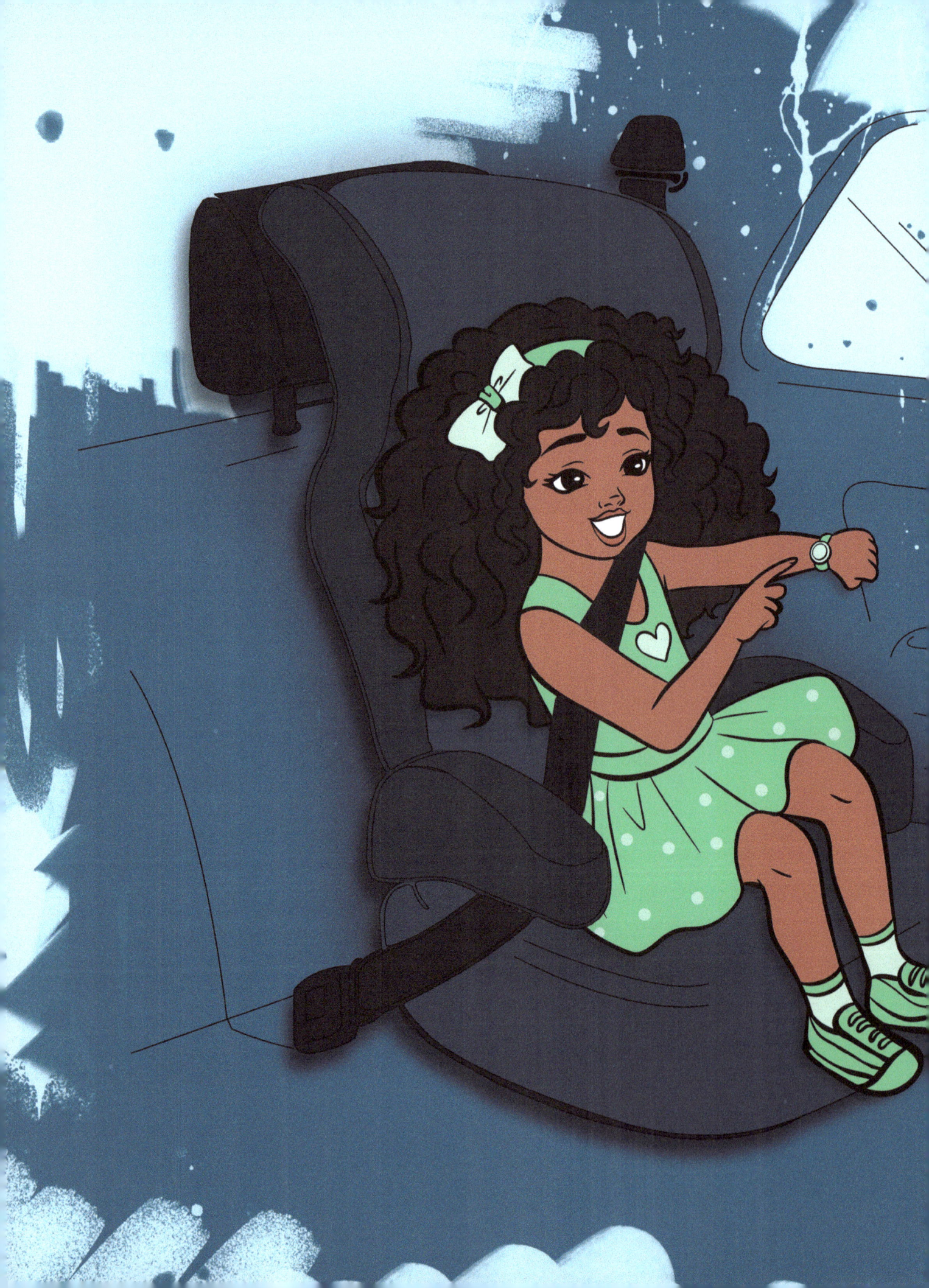

I buckled my seatbelt, and off we went.

Grandma and Dad sat in the front seats, and Mom and I sat in the back.

I looked at my watch. Now, you might be wondering why a little kid wears a watch. Well, like I said, I'm smart, so my parents got it for me for my birthday.

The ride was just thirty minutes.
But it seemed to take forever.

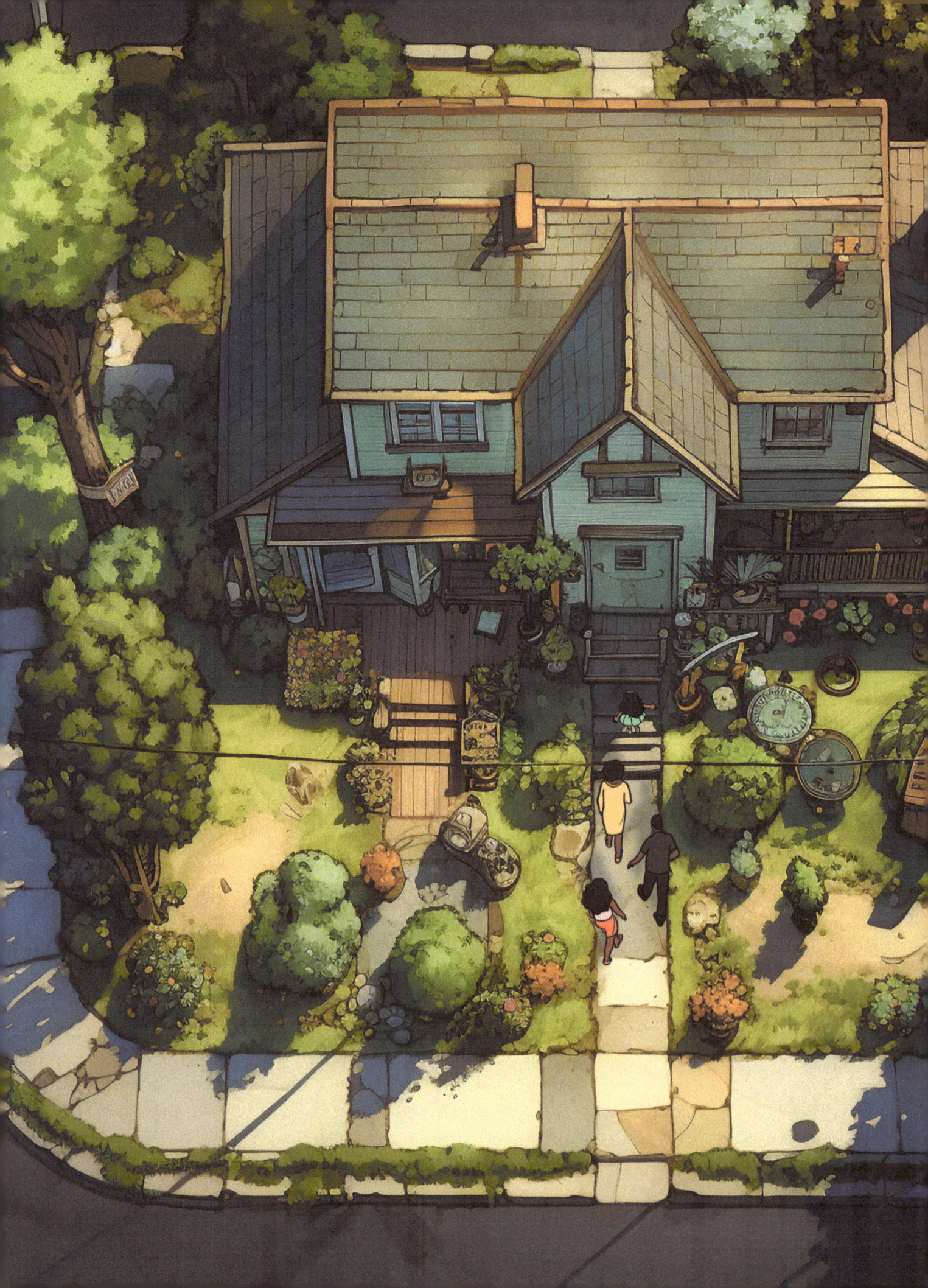

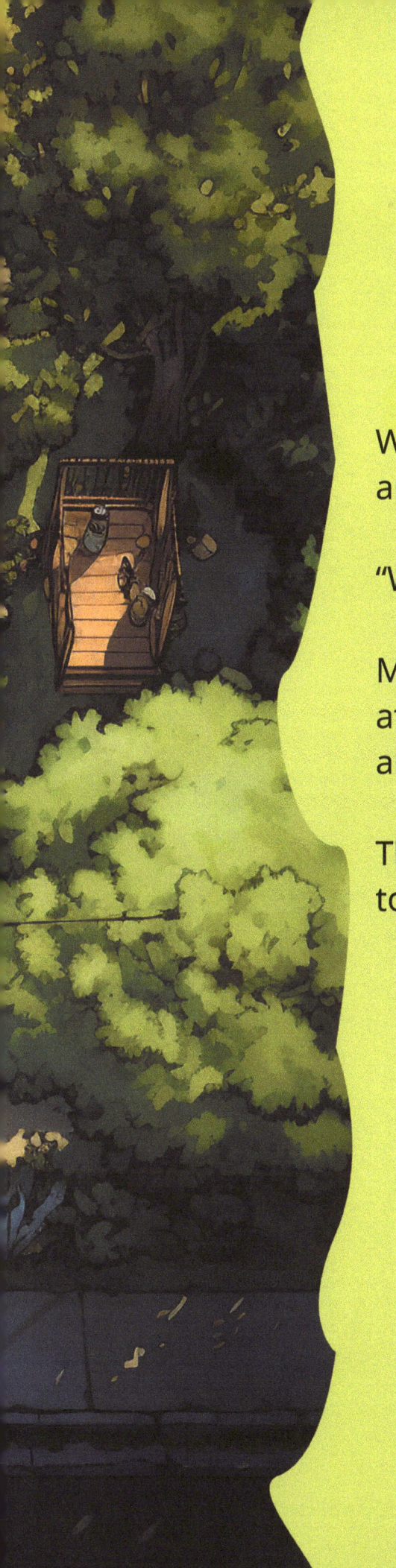

We arrived at Grandma's house, and Grandpa was not there.

"Where is Grandpa?"

Mom explained, "He is spending the night at a special home. You will see him bright and early Sunday morning."

That meant I had to wait another day to see Grandpa.

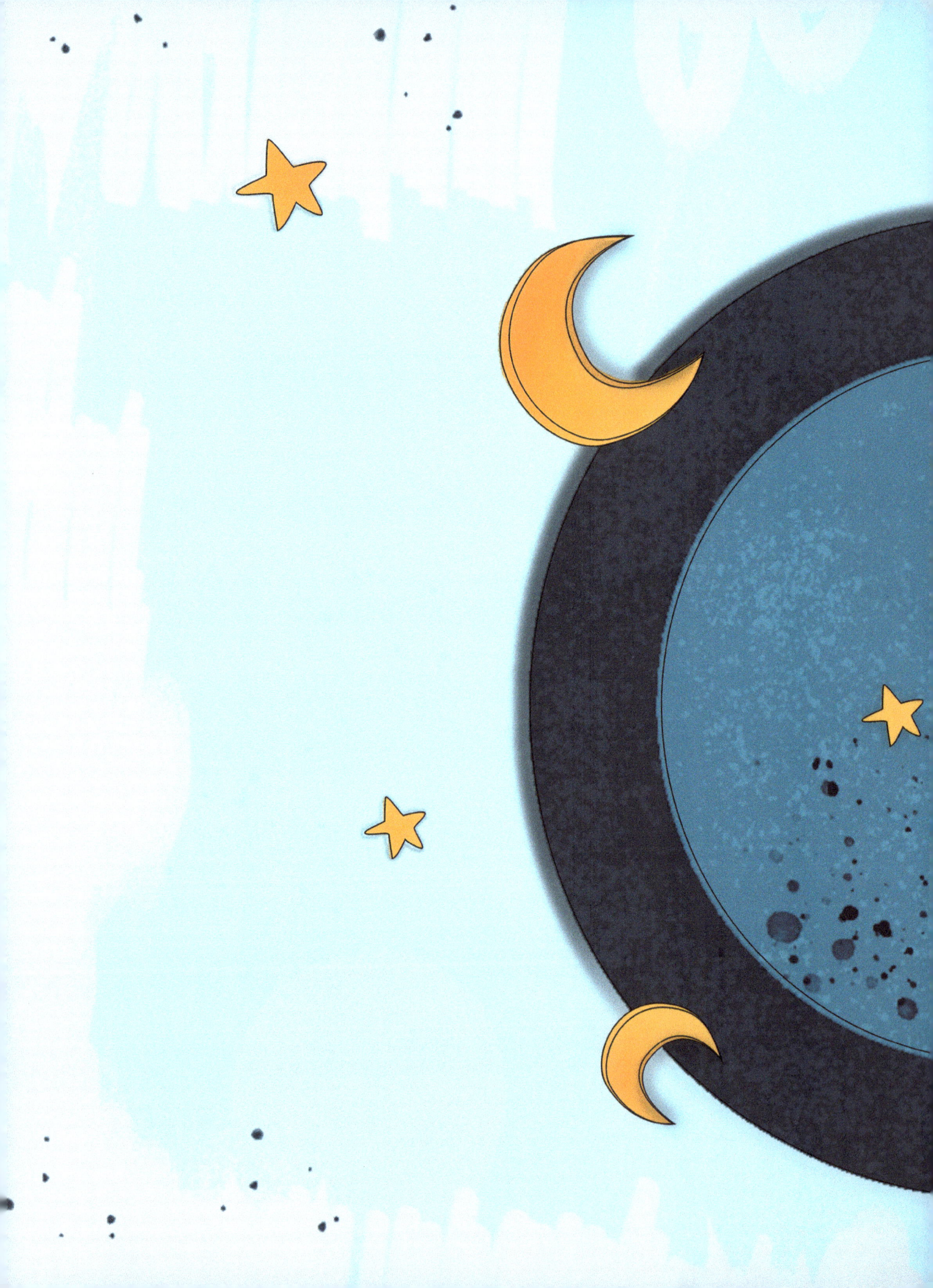

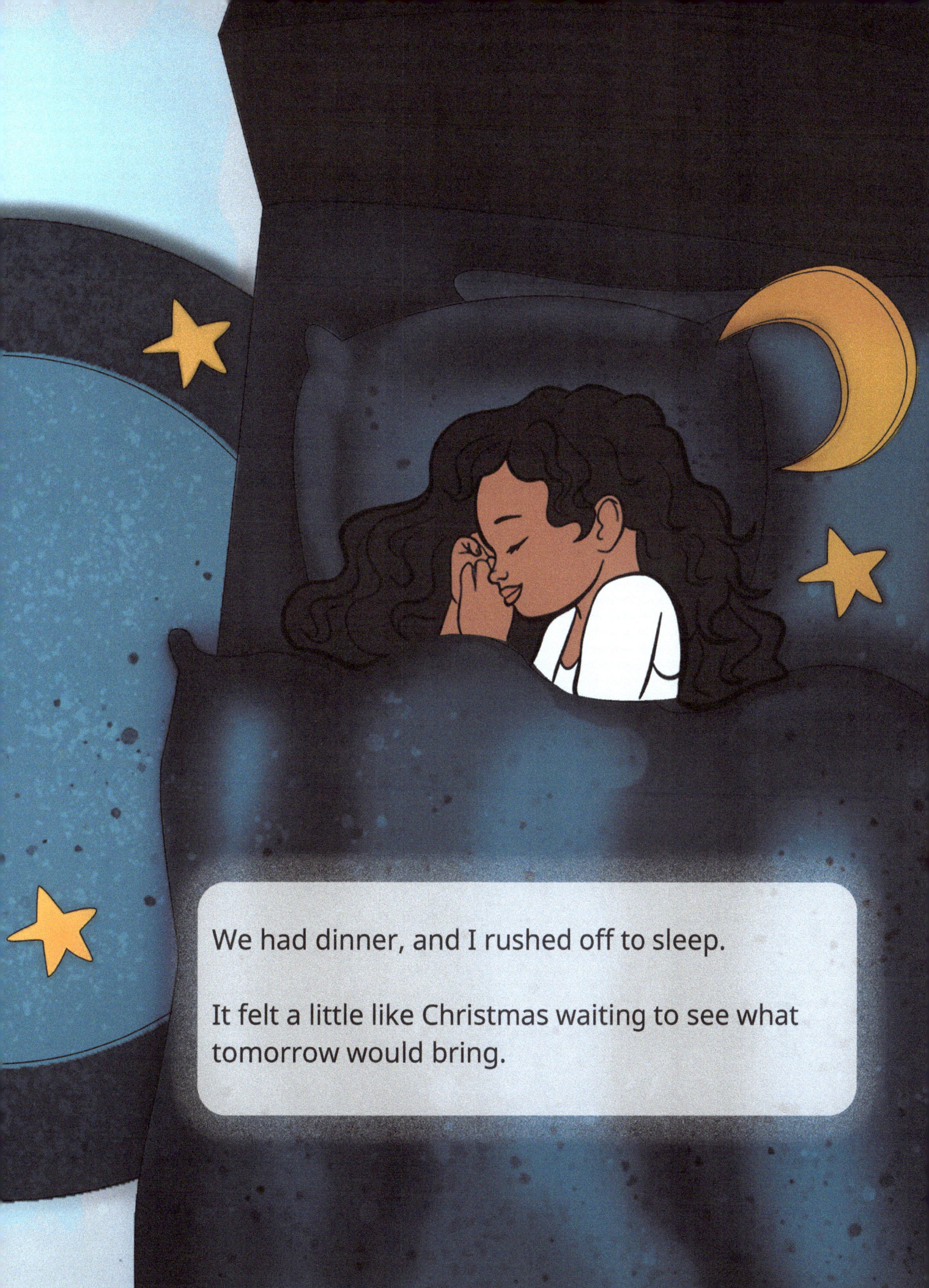

We had dinner, and I rushed off to sleep.

It felt a little like Christmas waiting to see what tomorrow would bring.

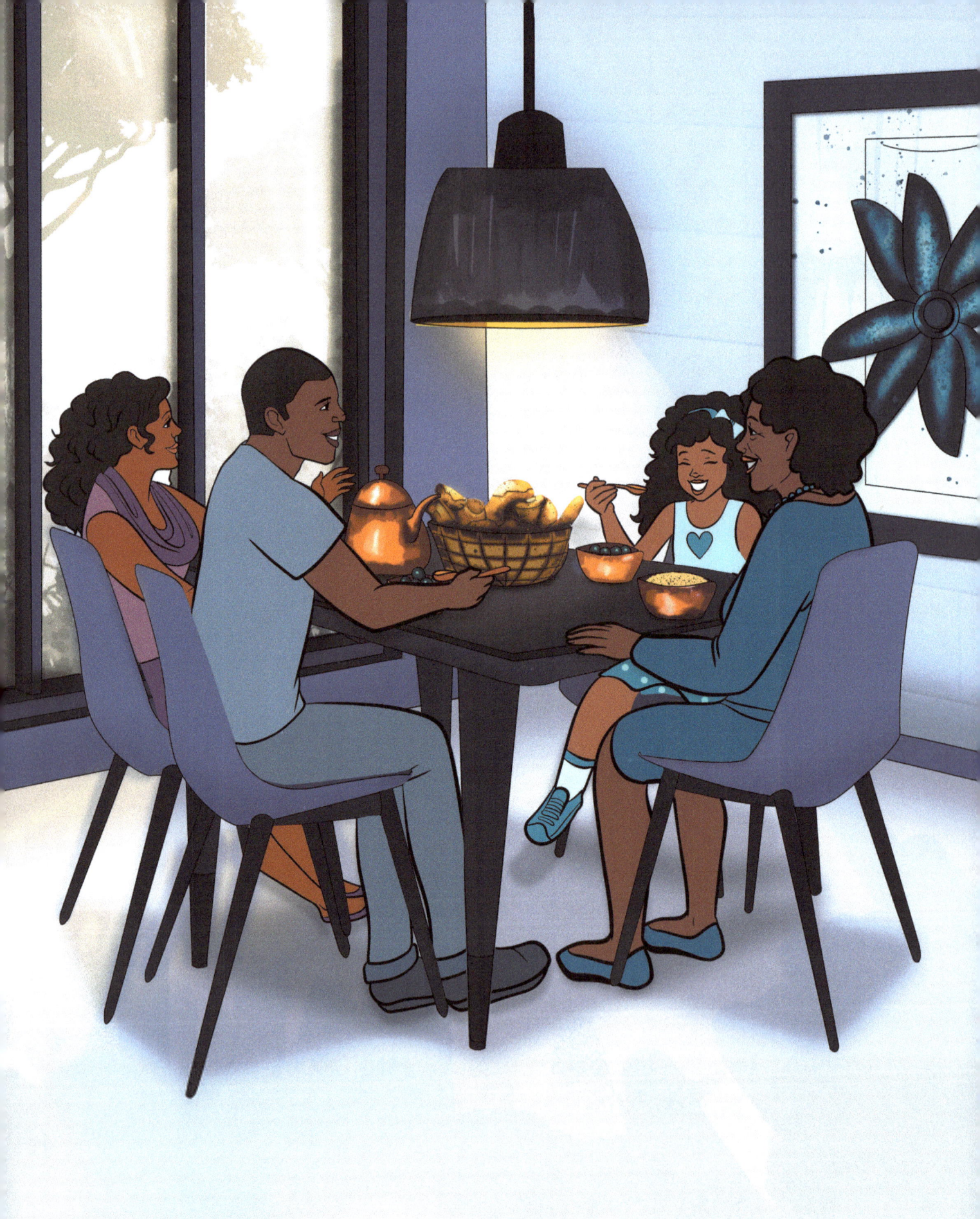

The next morning, we ate breakfast, and I finished really fast.

"Slow down, Charlotte. Are you in a hurry for something?"

"Yes!" I jiggled in my seat. "I want to go see Grandpa!"

Soon, everyone was finished eating breakfast, and we all loaded into Grandma's car.

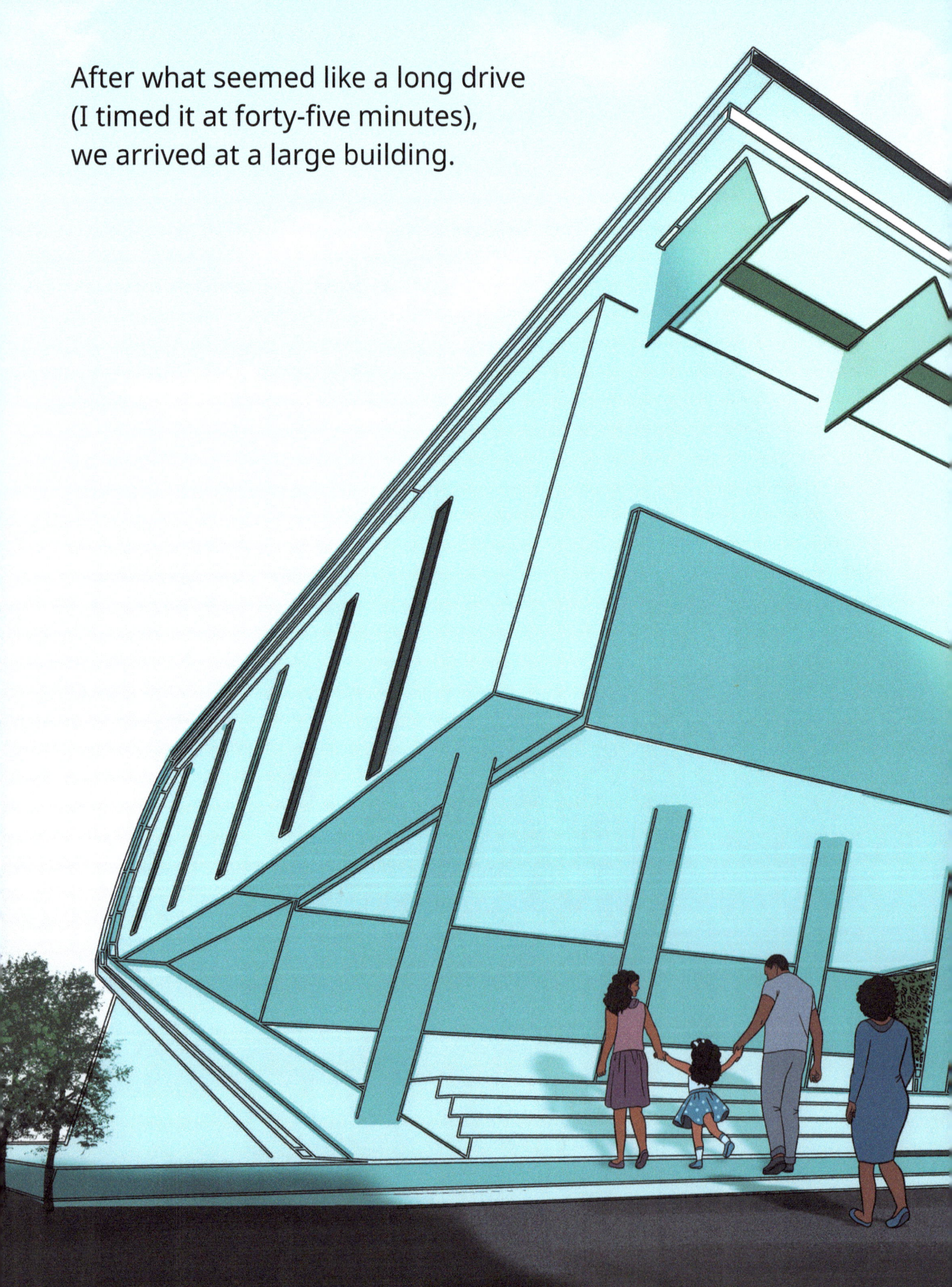
After what seemed like a long drive (I timed it at forty-five minutes), we arrived at a large building.

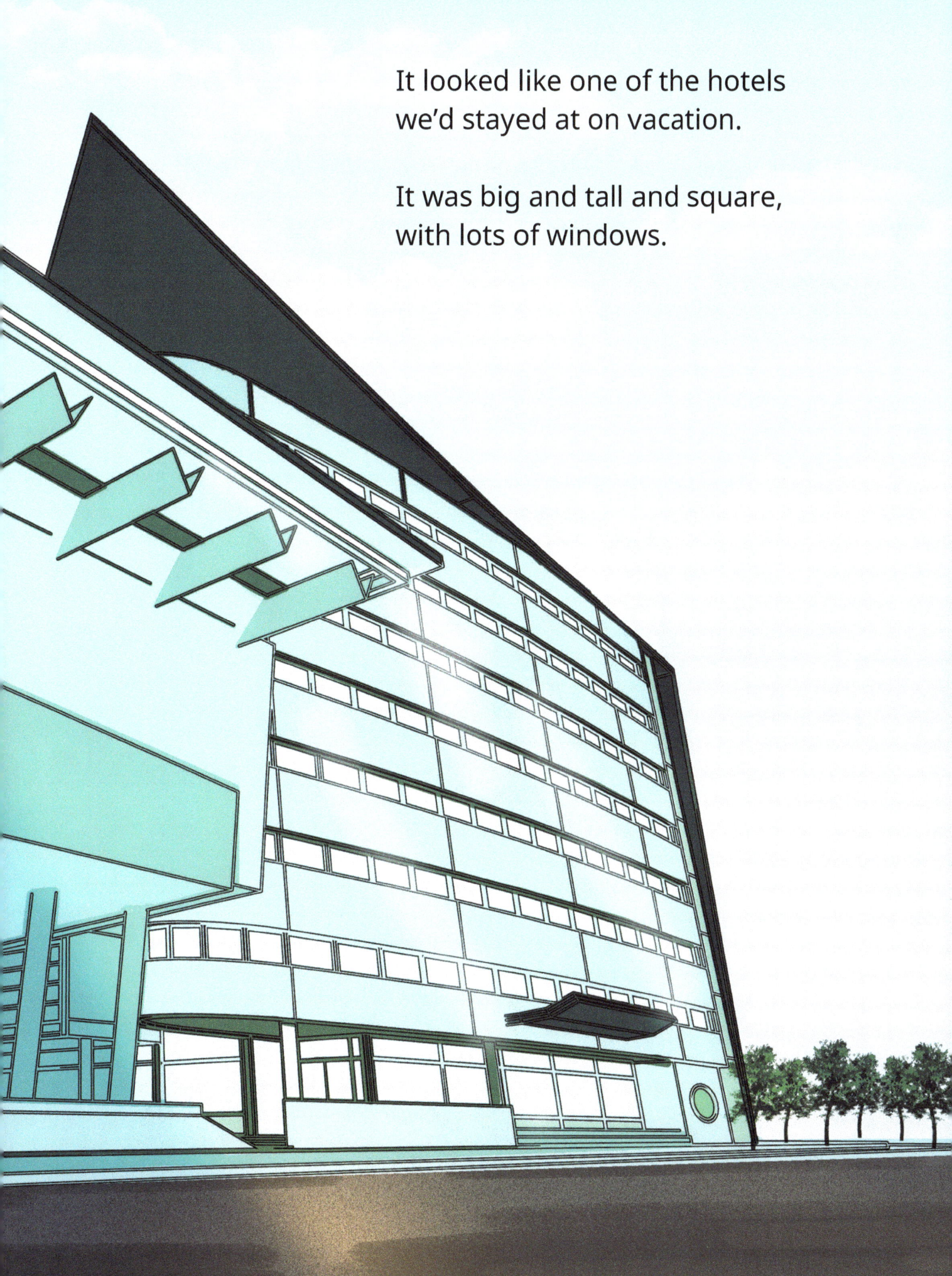

When we walked in through the big double doors,
the first thing I noticed was a fireplace,
but I think it was one of those fake ones that looked real.
There were chairs next to it with high backs.

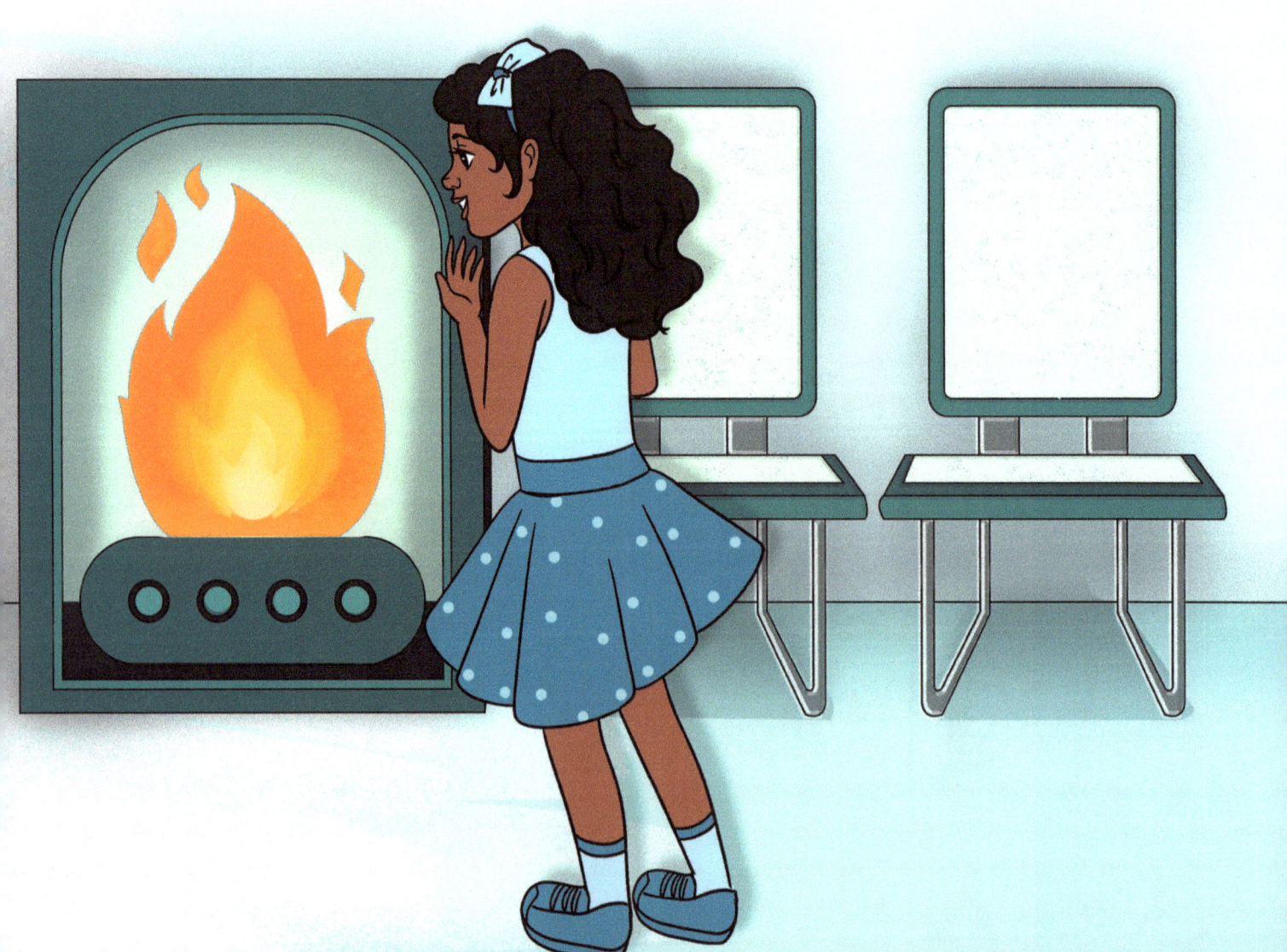

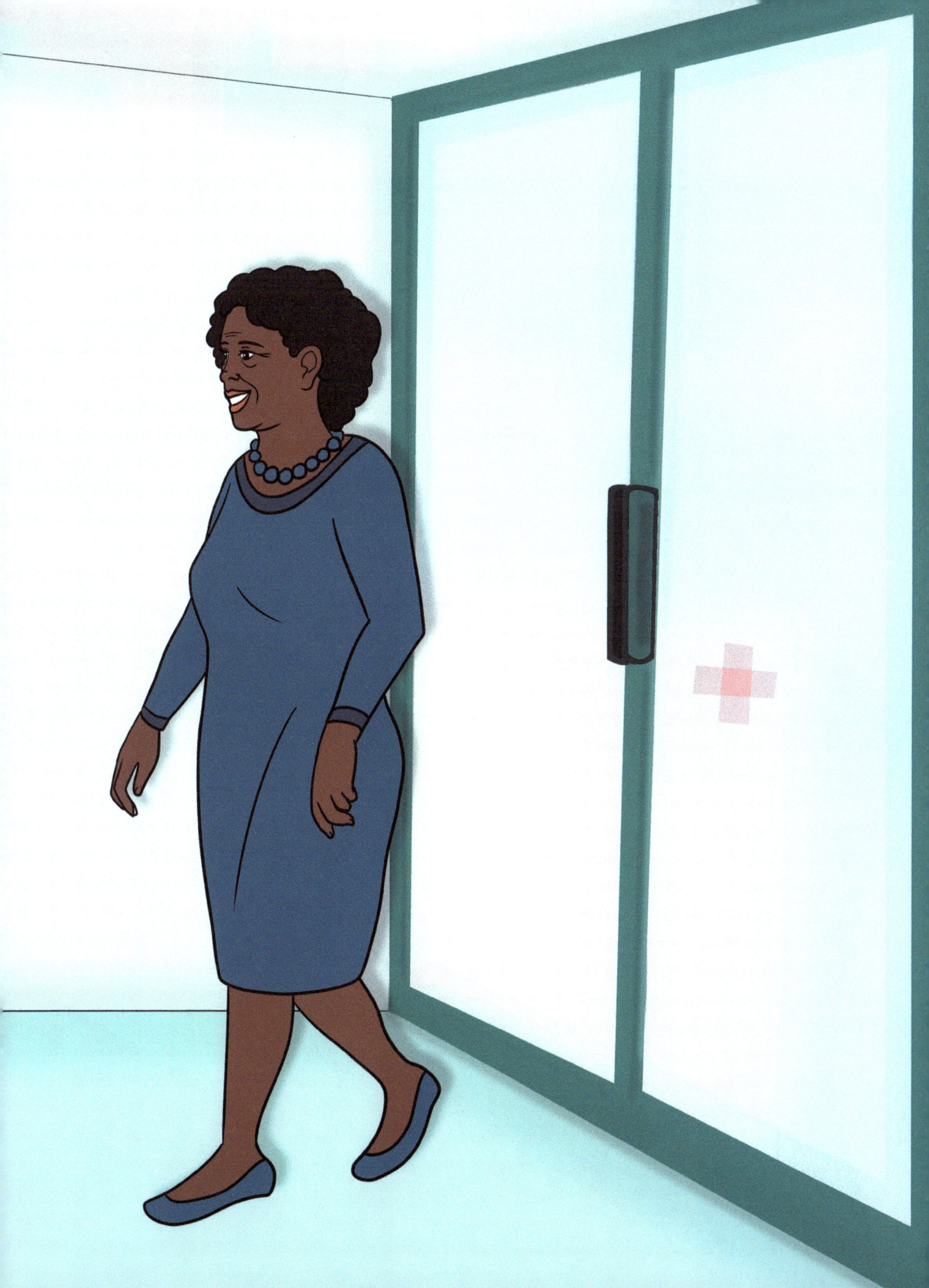

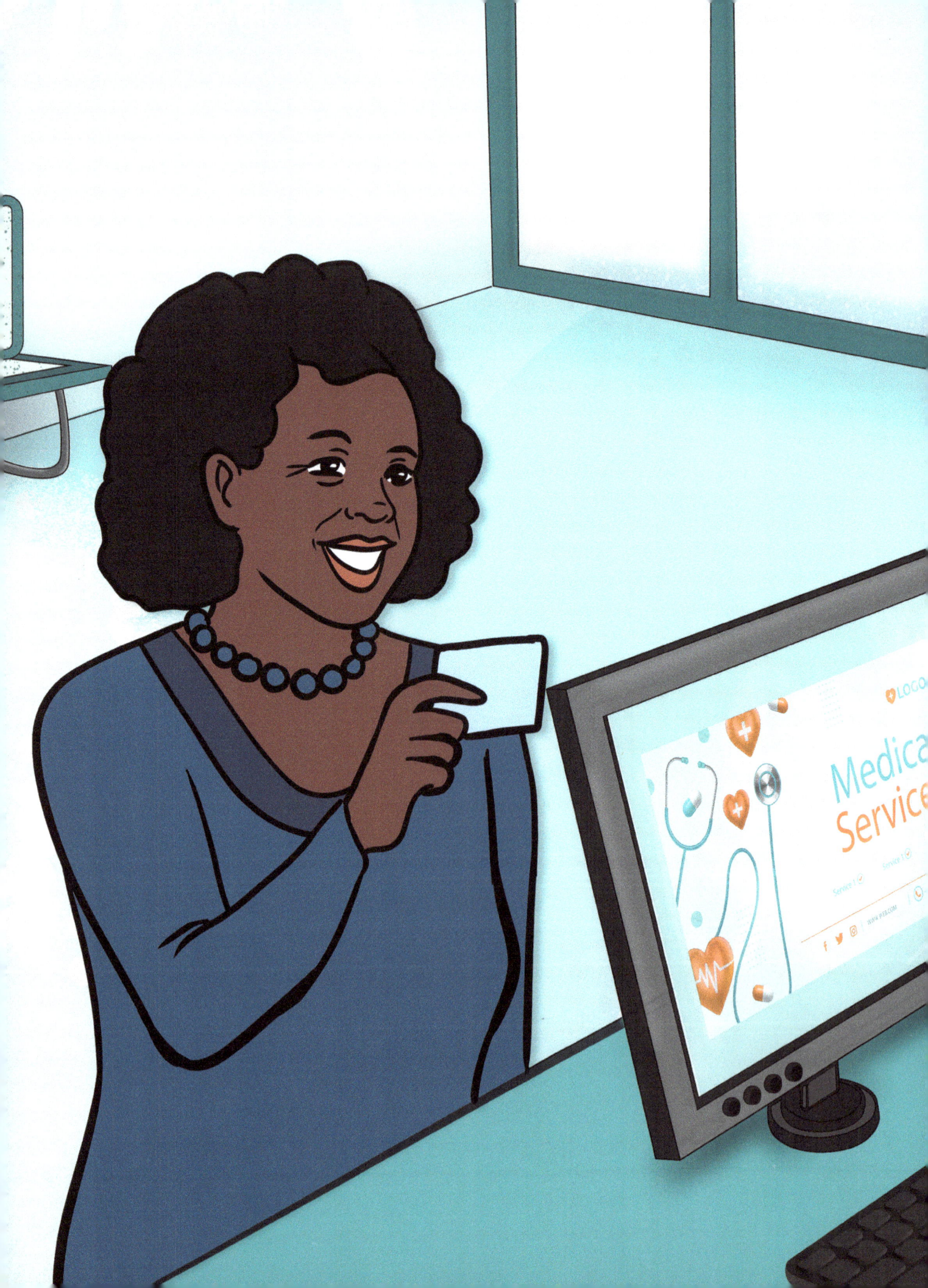

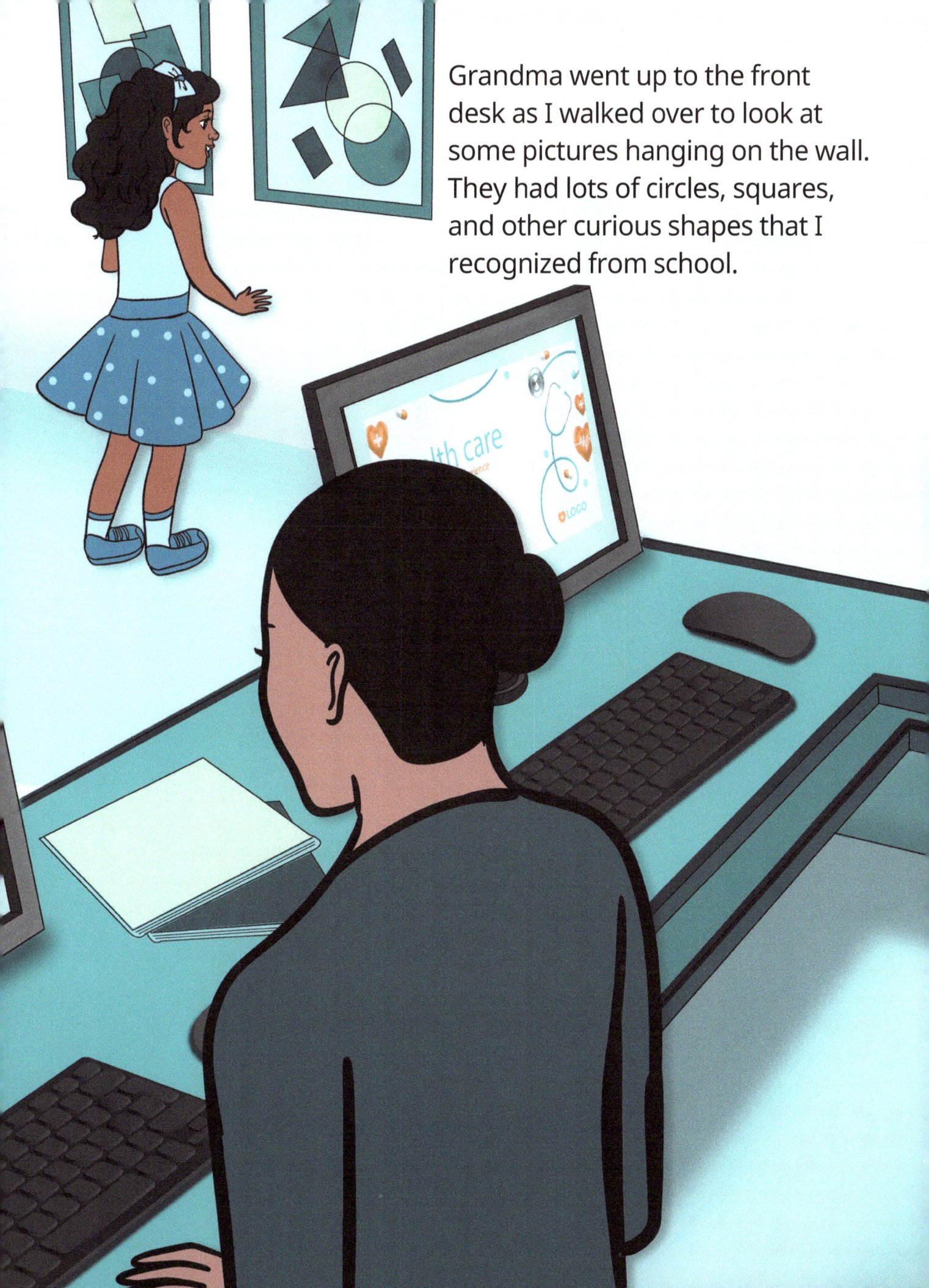

Grandma went up to the front desk as I walked over to look at some pictures hanging on the wall. They had lots of circles, squares, and other curious shapes that I recognized from school.

But before I could get a good look, Dad called me over, and a lady in a green suit guided us into another room.

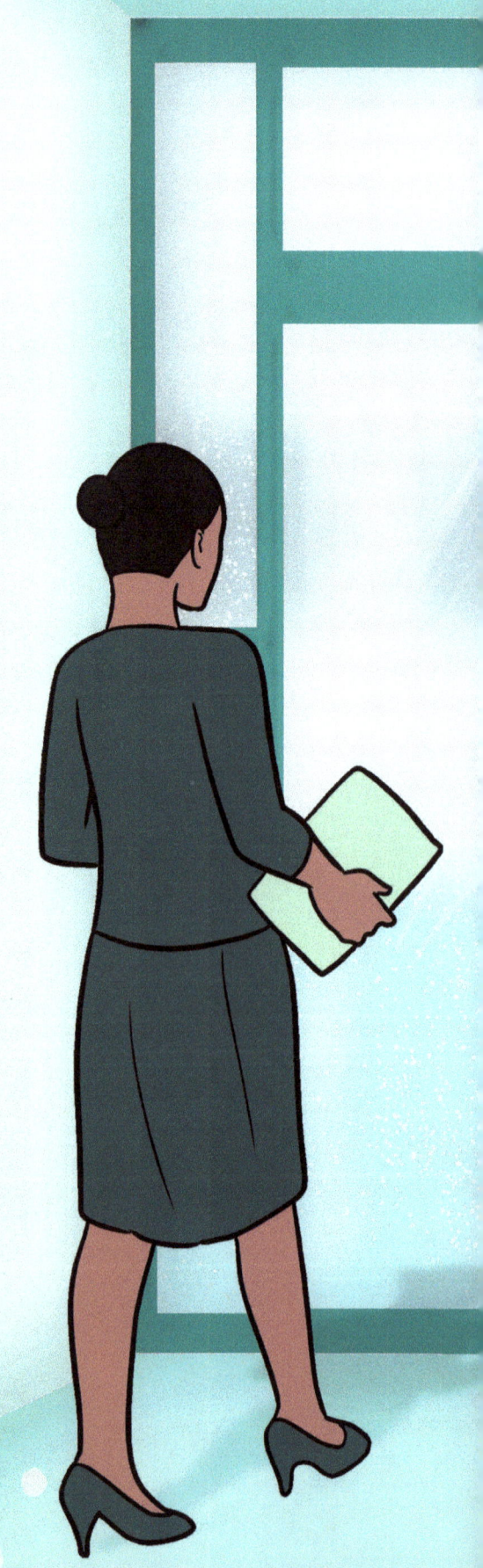

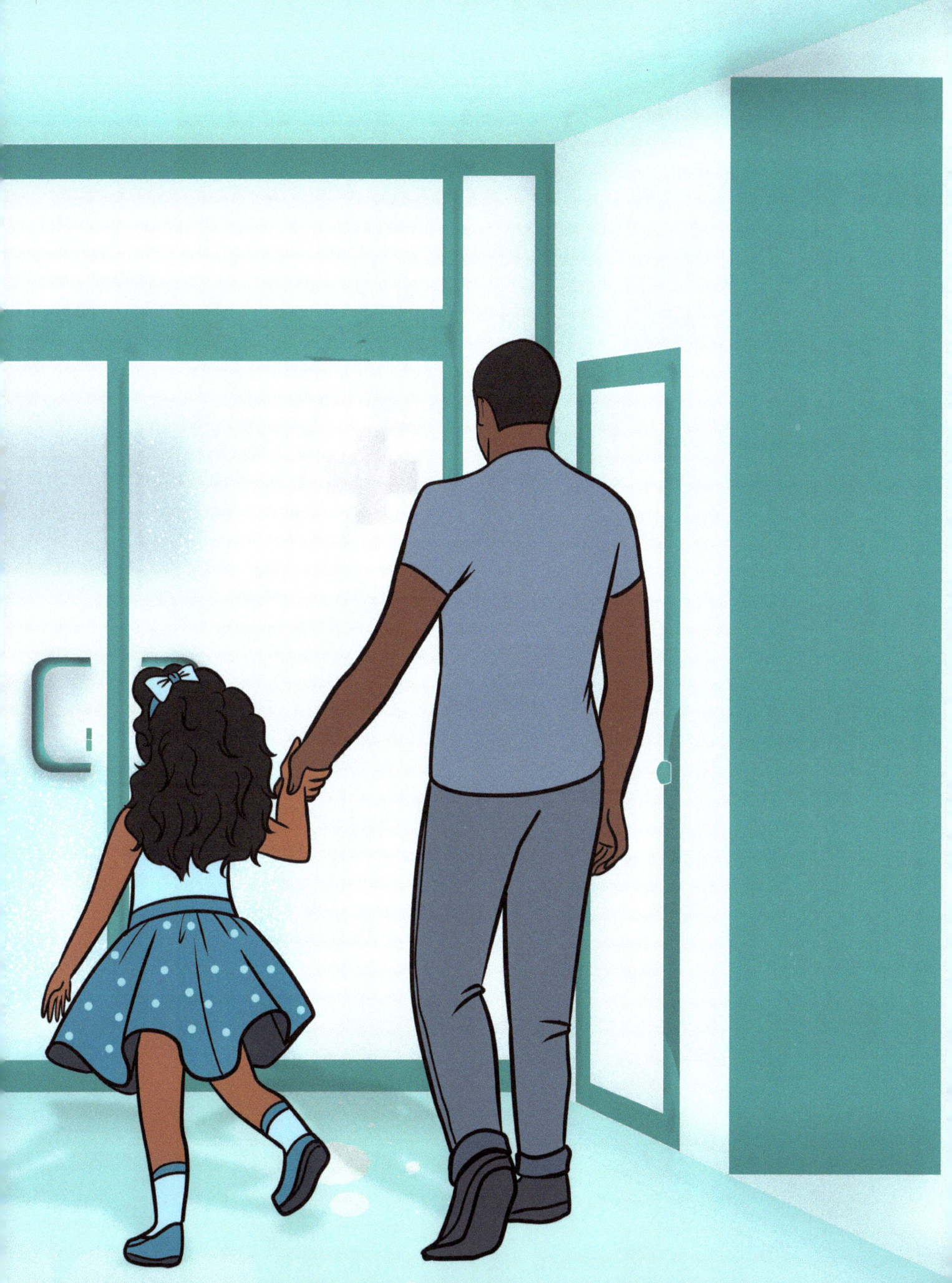

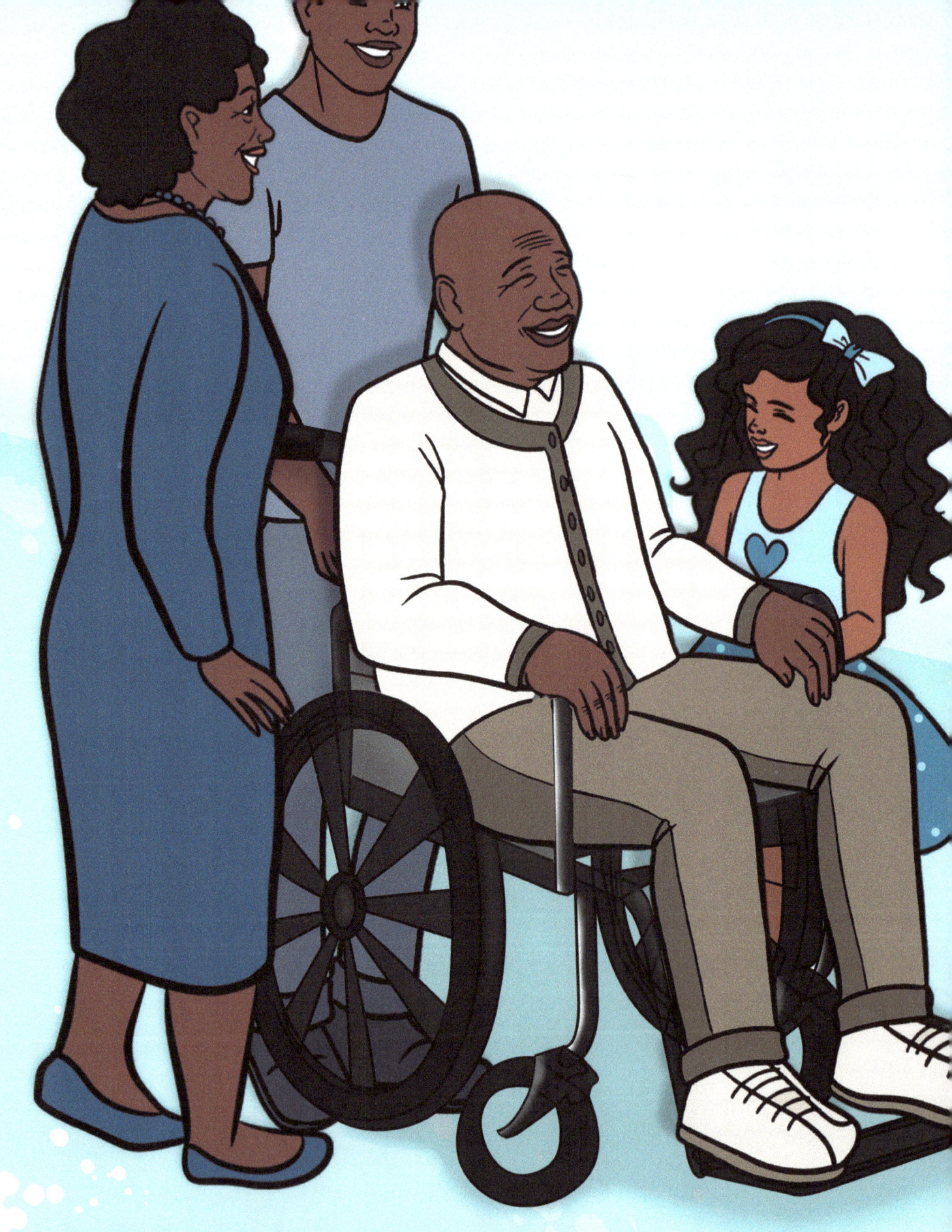

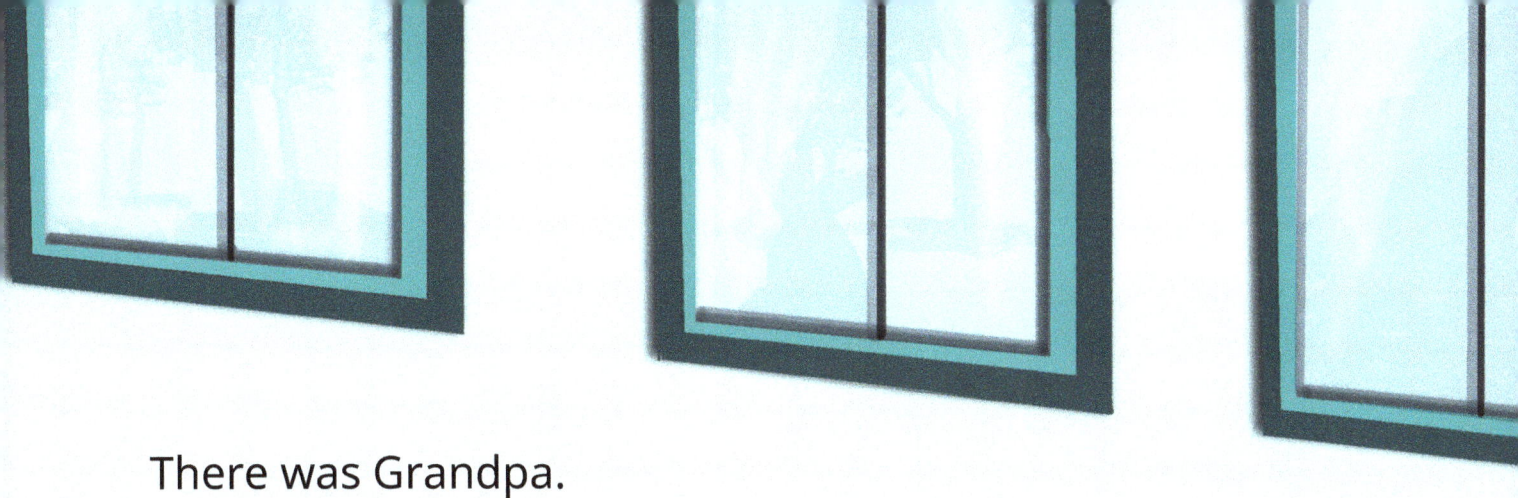

There was Grandpa.

He was in a wheelchair. But that didn't matter to me.
It was my grandpa. I ran to him and gave him a big hug.

He hugged me back with a big smile and the deep laughter
I had known all my life.

Then he said, "And who are you, little girl?" Pointing at
Grandma, he added, "And who is that pretty lady with you?"

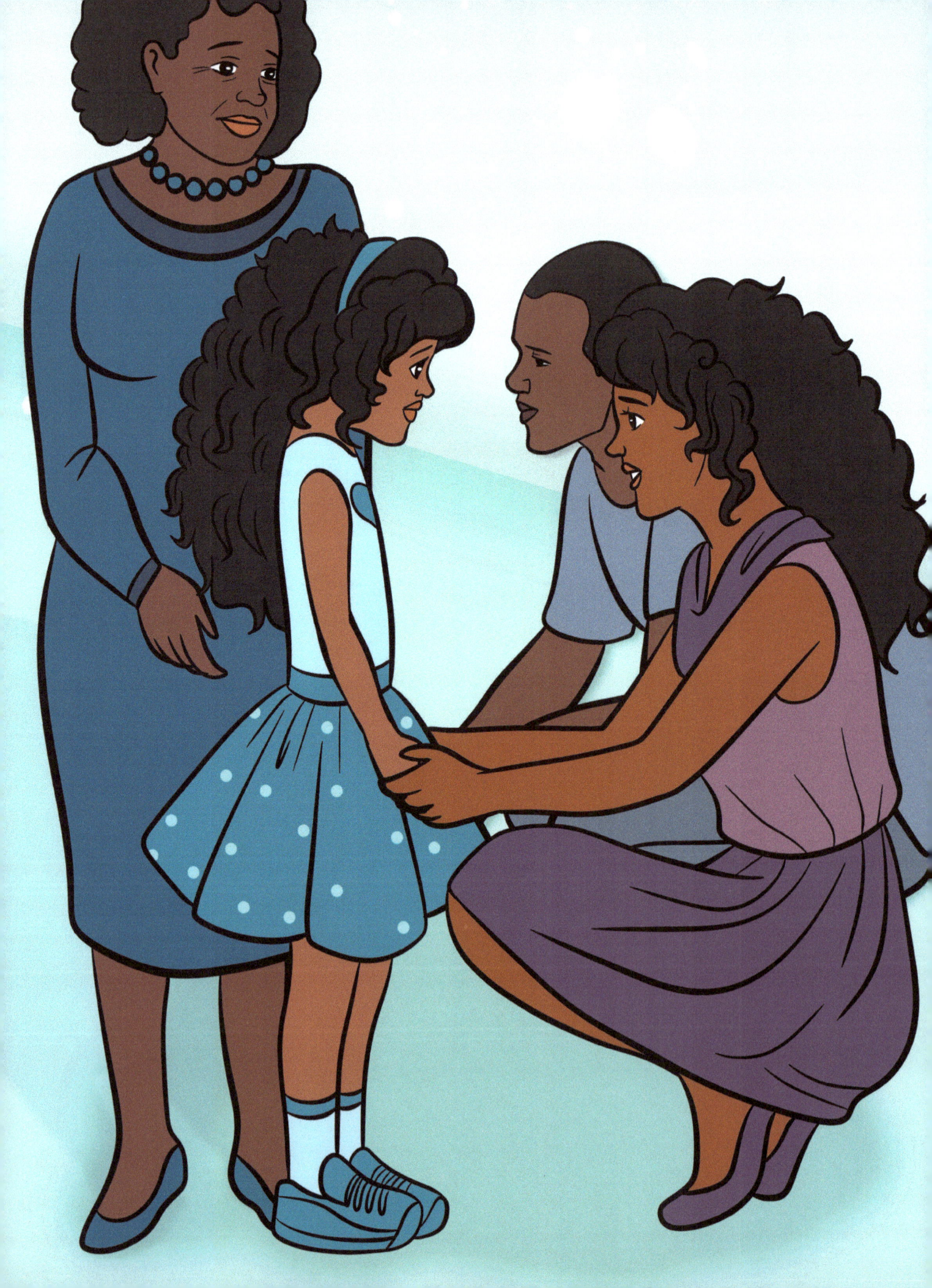

"Mom, Dad, Grandpa forgot my name!"

Mom and Dad kneeled in front of me.

Grandma stood silently behind them, occasionally waving at hospital type folks as they passed.

Dad said, in a quiet but strong voice,
"Grandpa has Alzheimer's."

"What's that?" I asked.
"Is it like a cold or something?"

"No, Charlotte, it's not like a cold.
It will not go away. Grandpa won't be able to remember things like he used to."

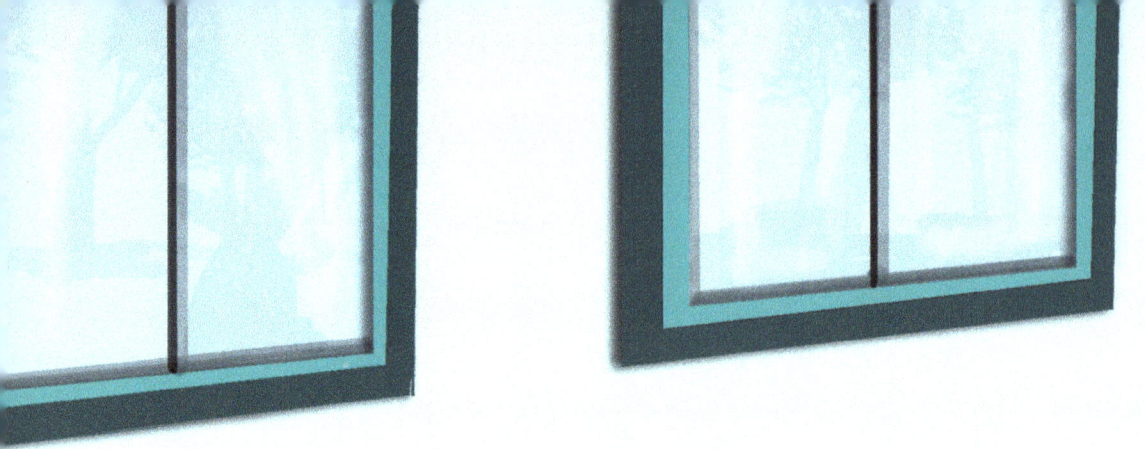

I stood next to Grandpa, and he held my hand.
He continued to look at Grandma with a loving smile.

We drove back to Grandma's house in silence.
No one seemed to want to talk.
The airplane ride home was not any better.

What was this Alzheimer's?
I wondered.

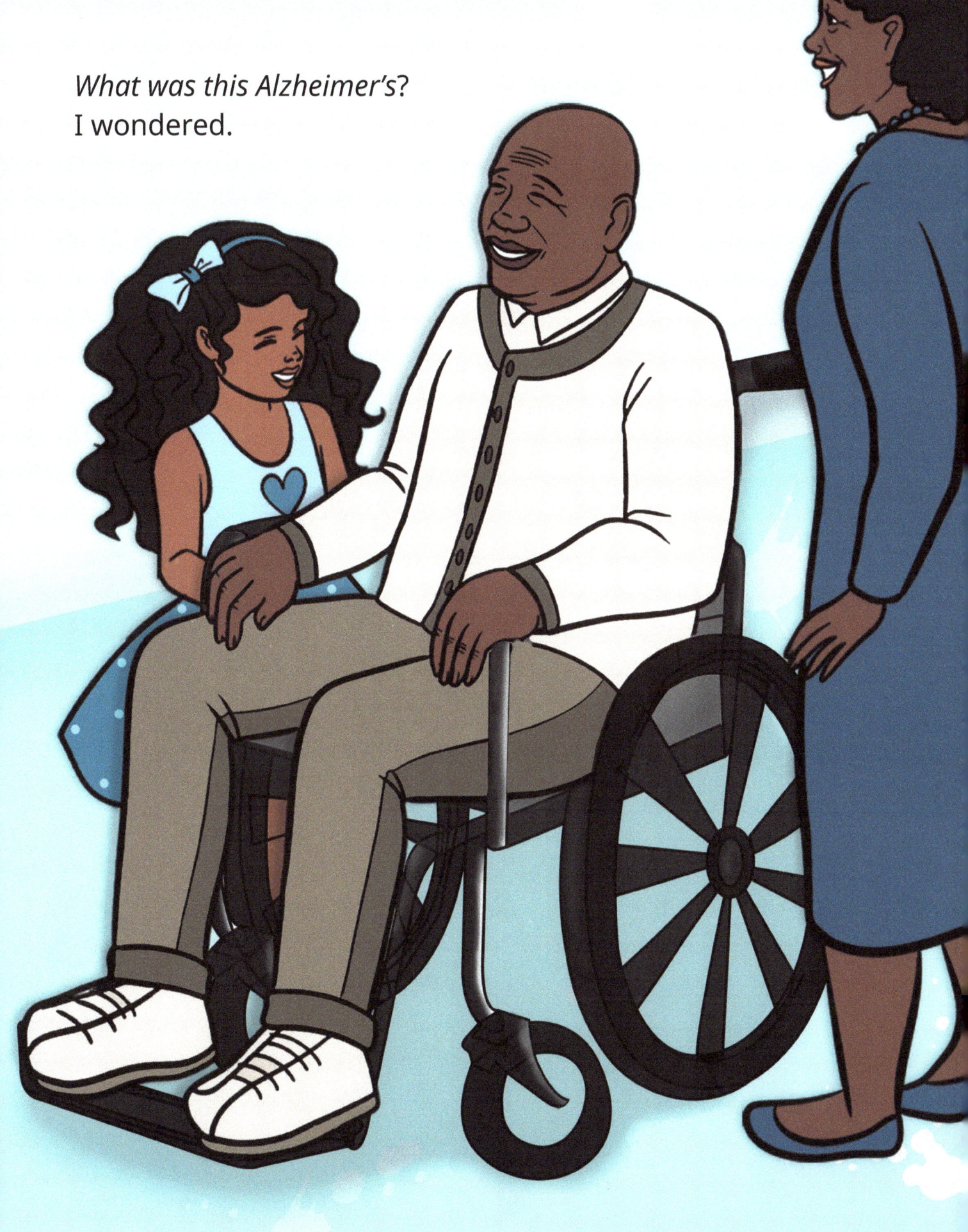

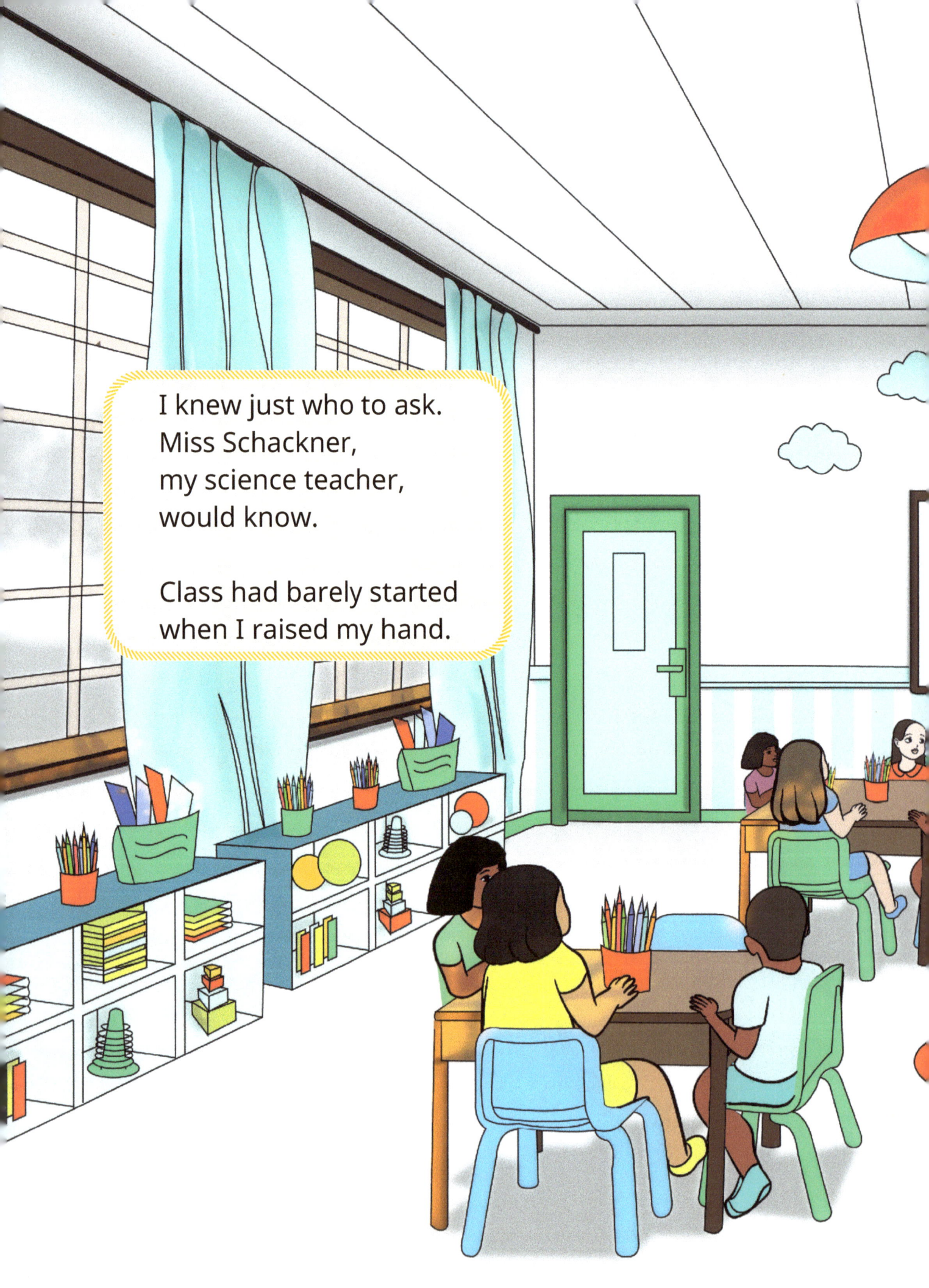

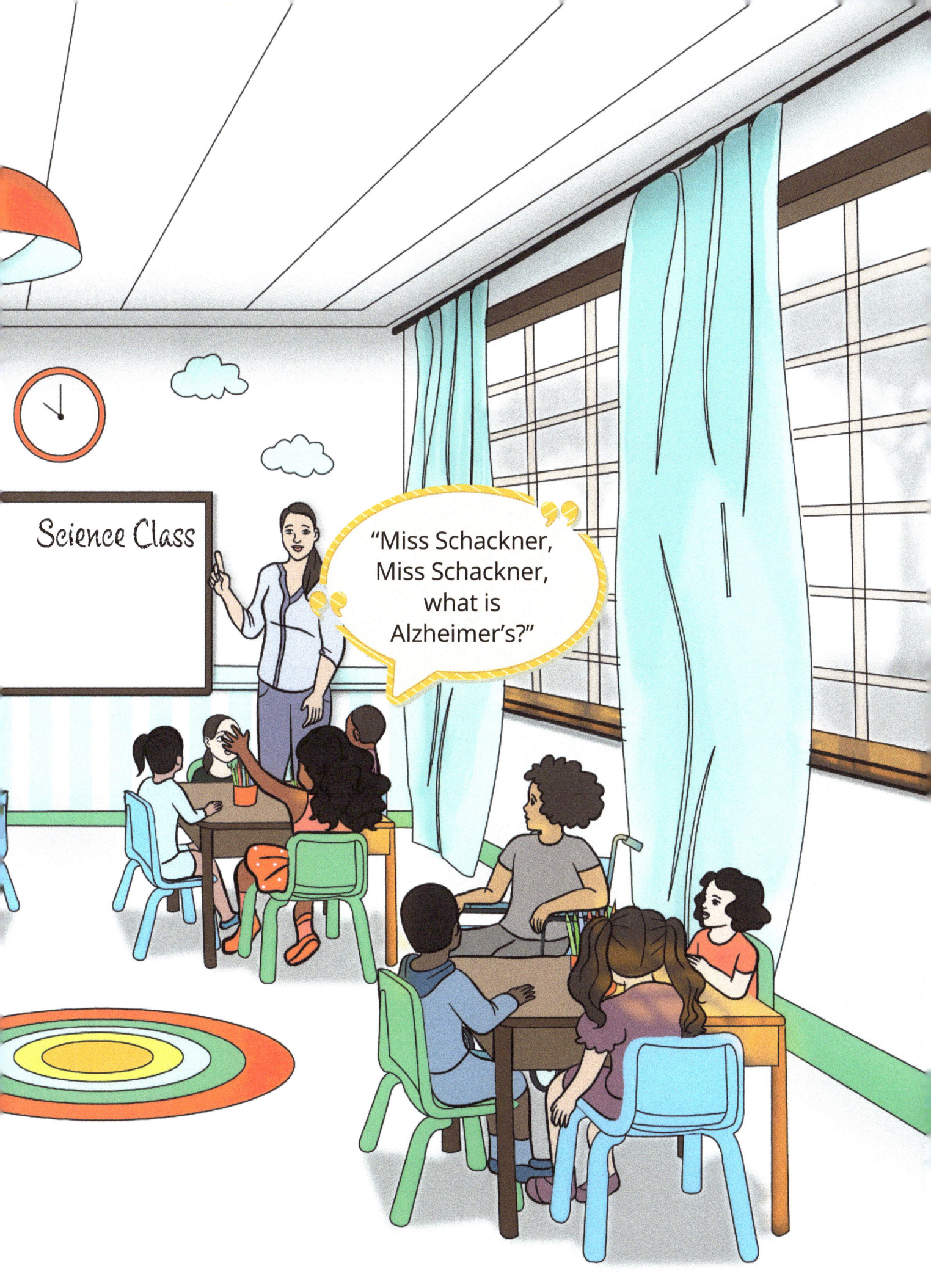

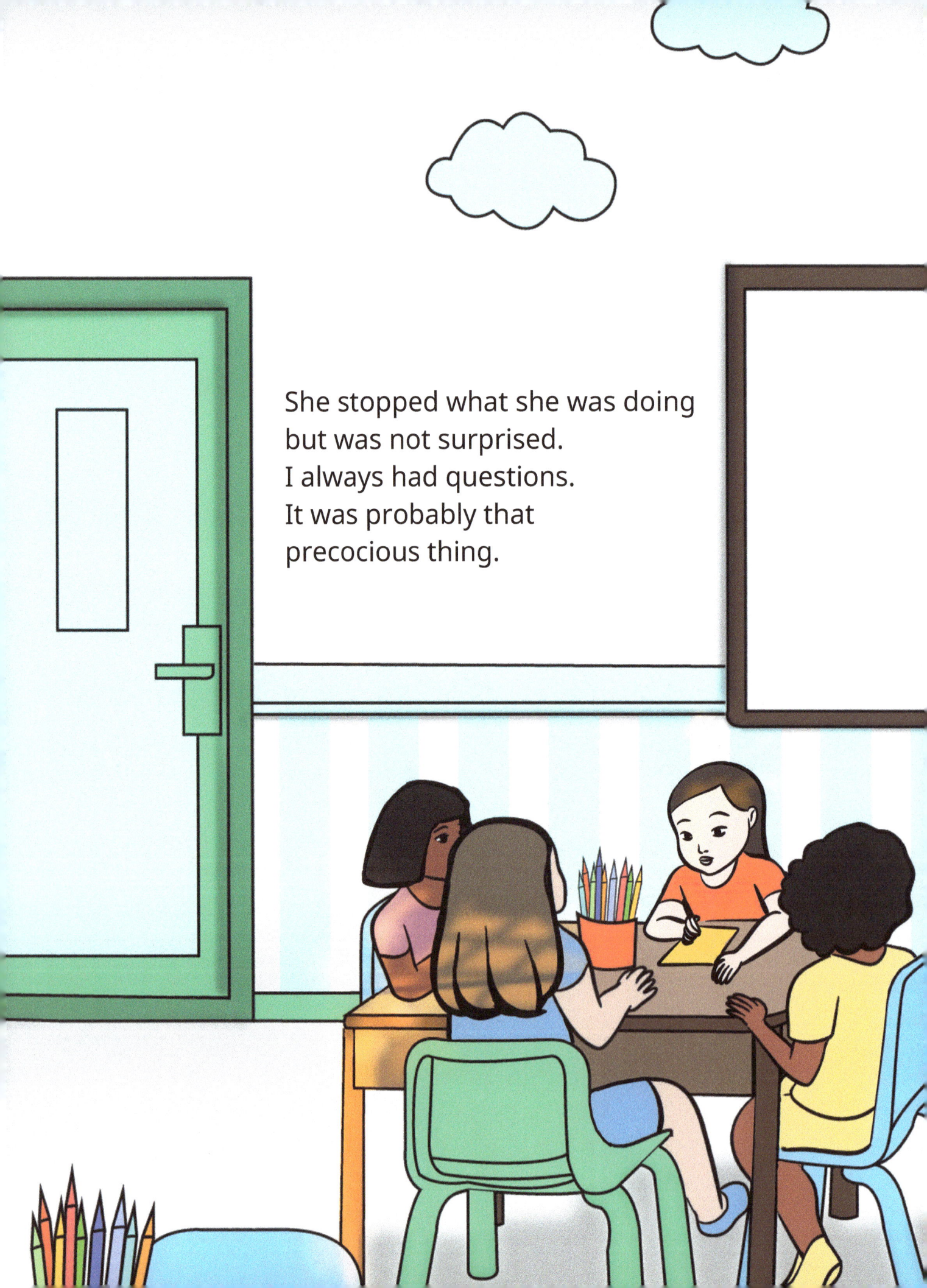

She stopped what she was doing but was not surprised.
I always had questions.
It was probably that precocious thing.

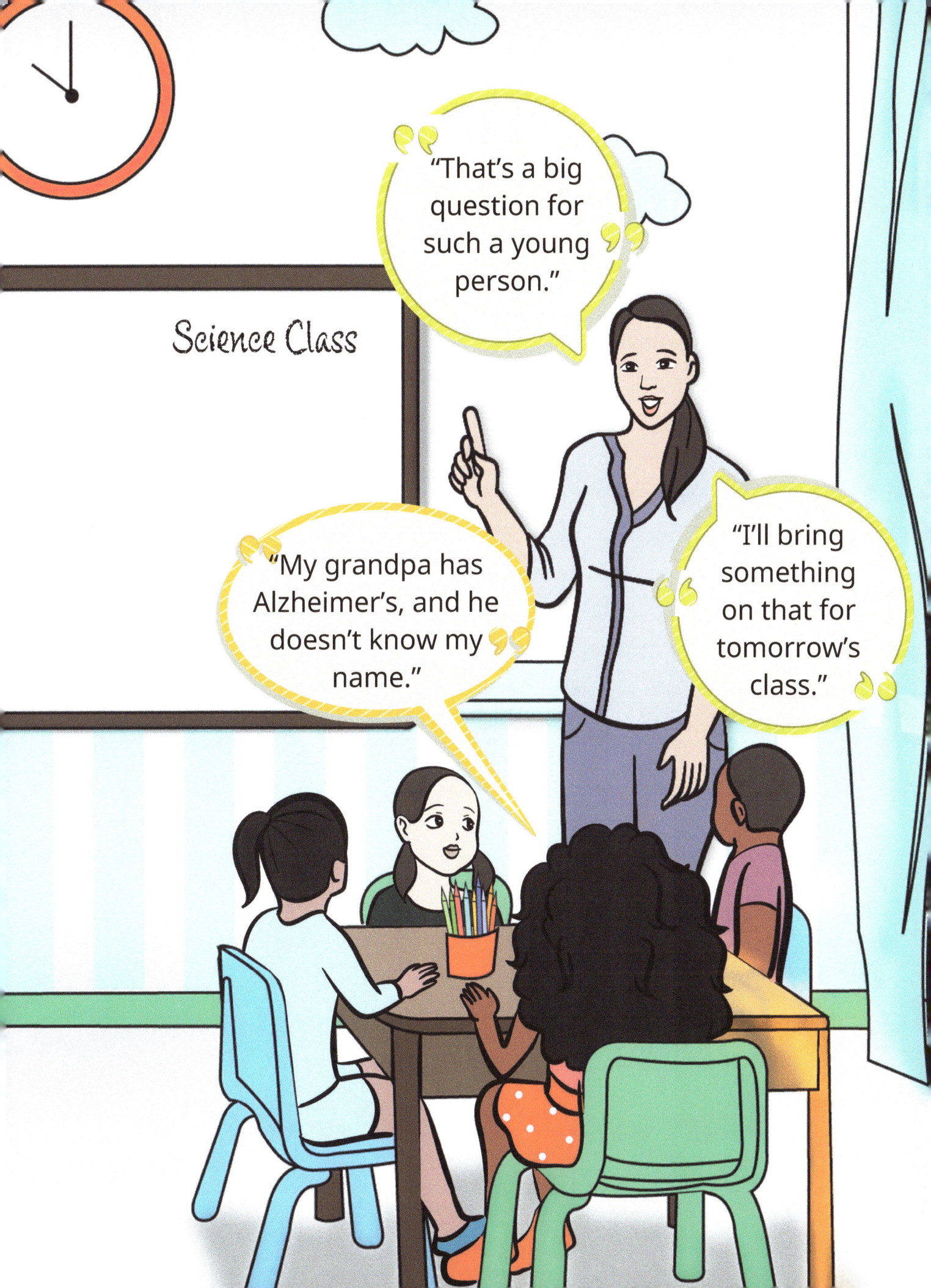

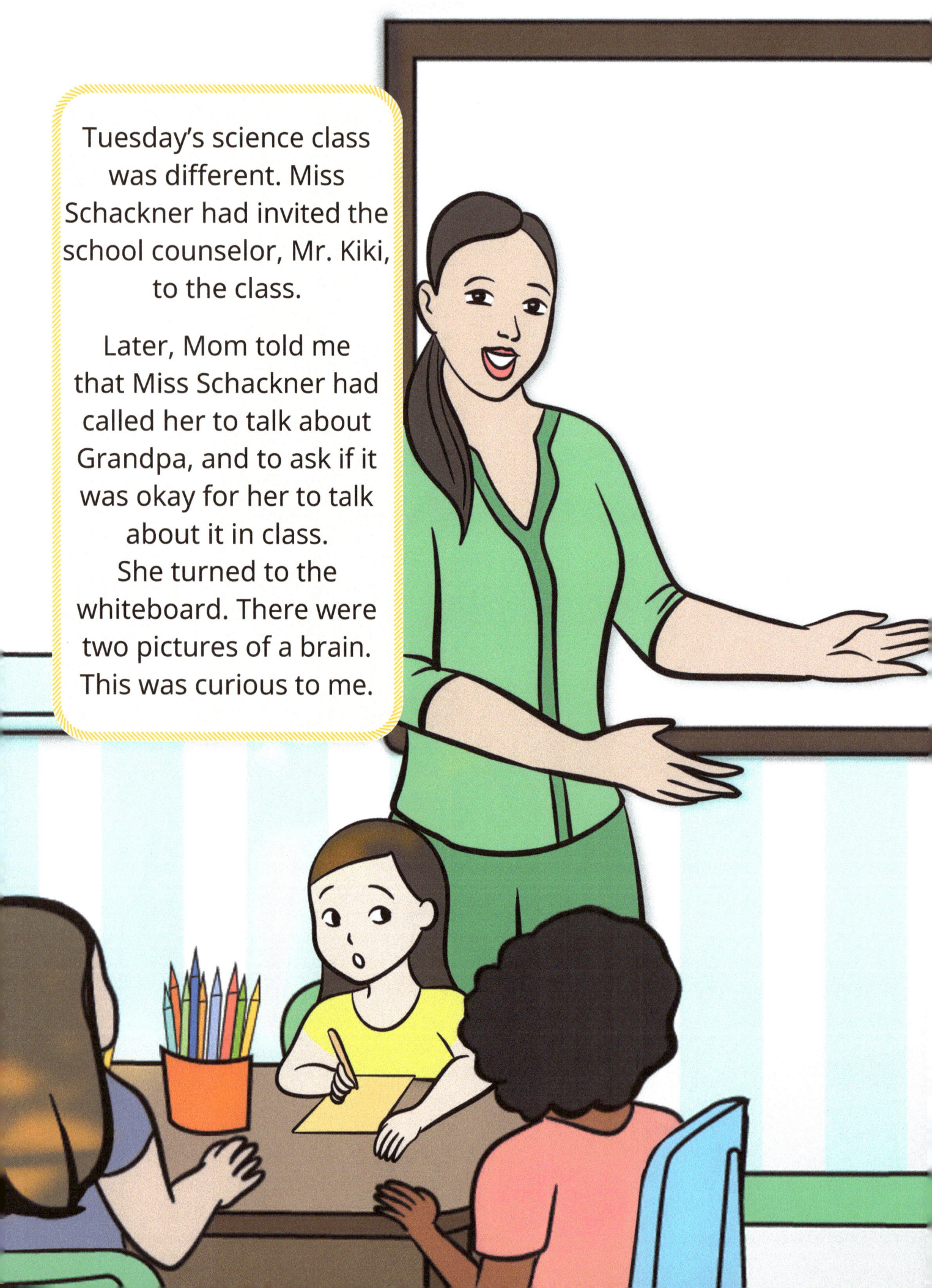

Tuesday's science class was different. Miss Schackner had invited the school counselor, Mr. Kiki, to the class.

Later, Mom told me that Miss Schackner had called her to talk about Grandpa, and to ask if it was okay for her to talk about it in class.
She turned to the whiteboard. There were two pictures of a brain. This was curious to me.

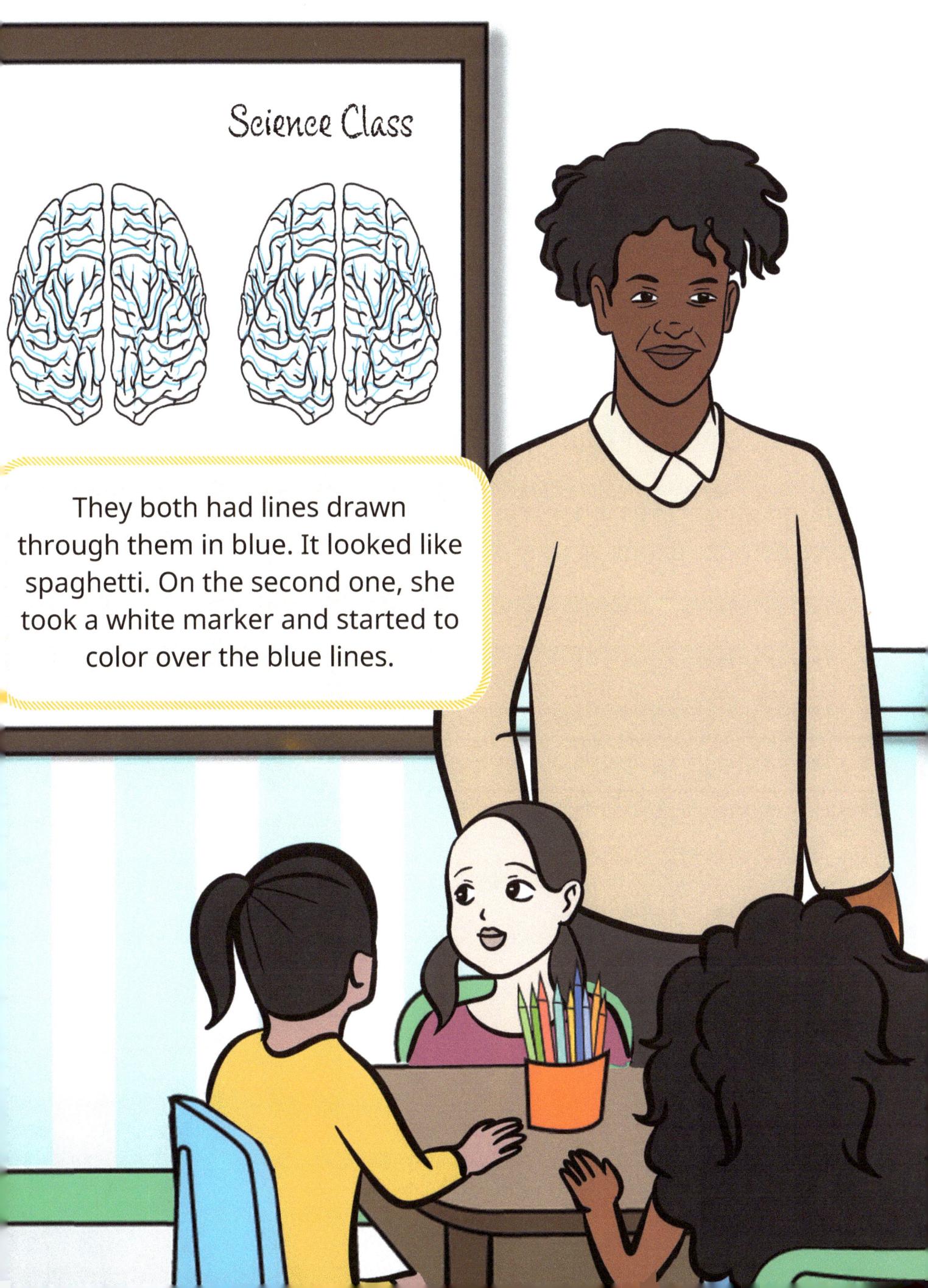

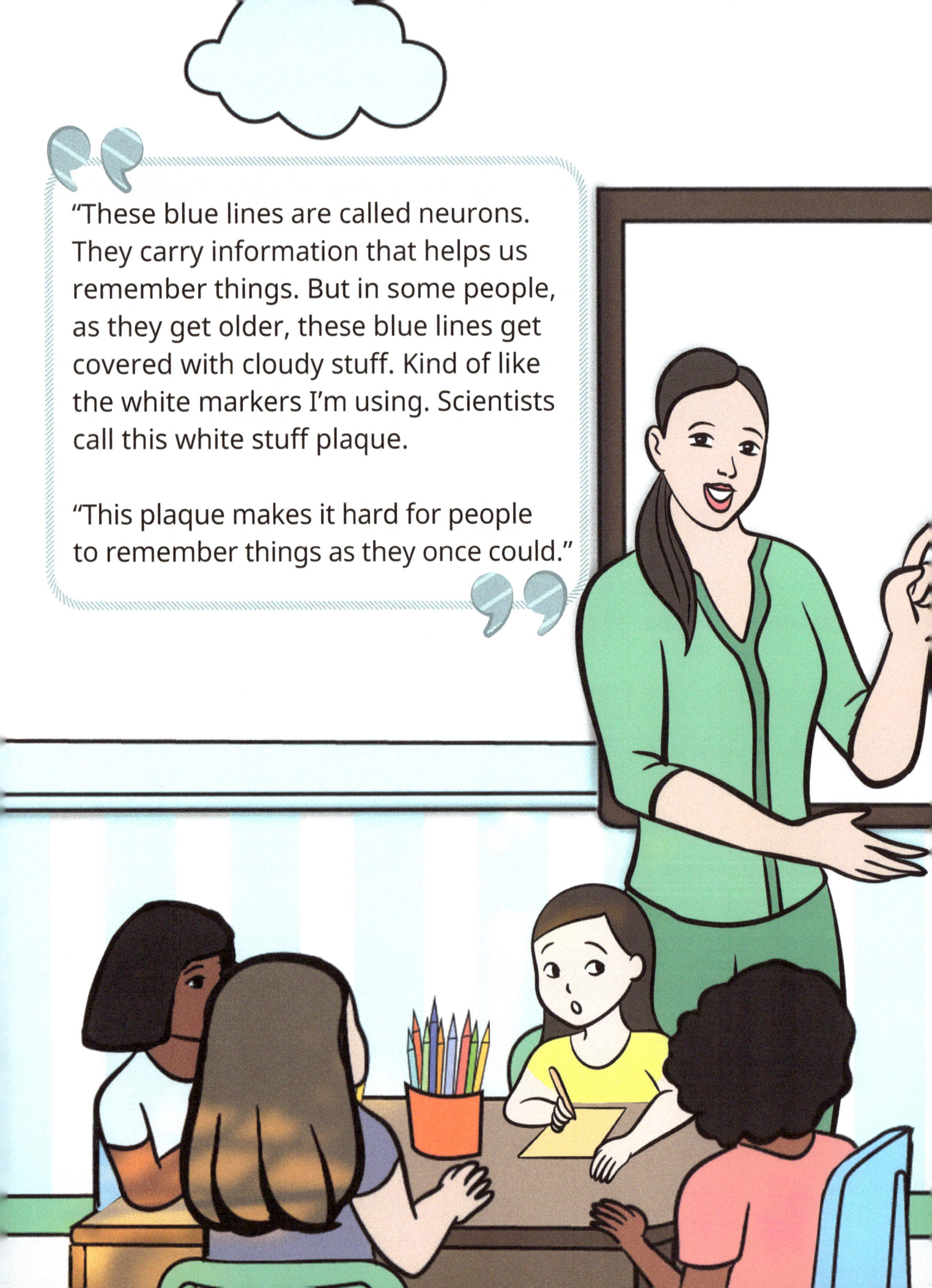

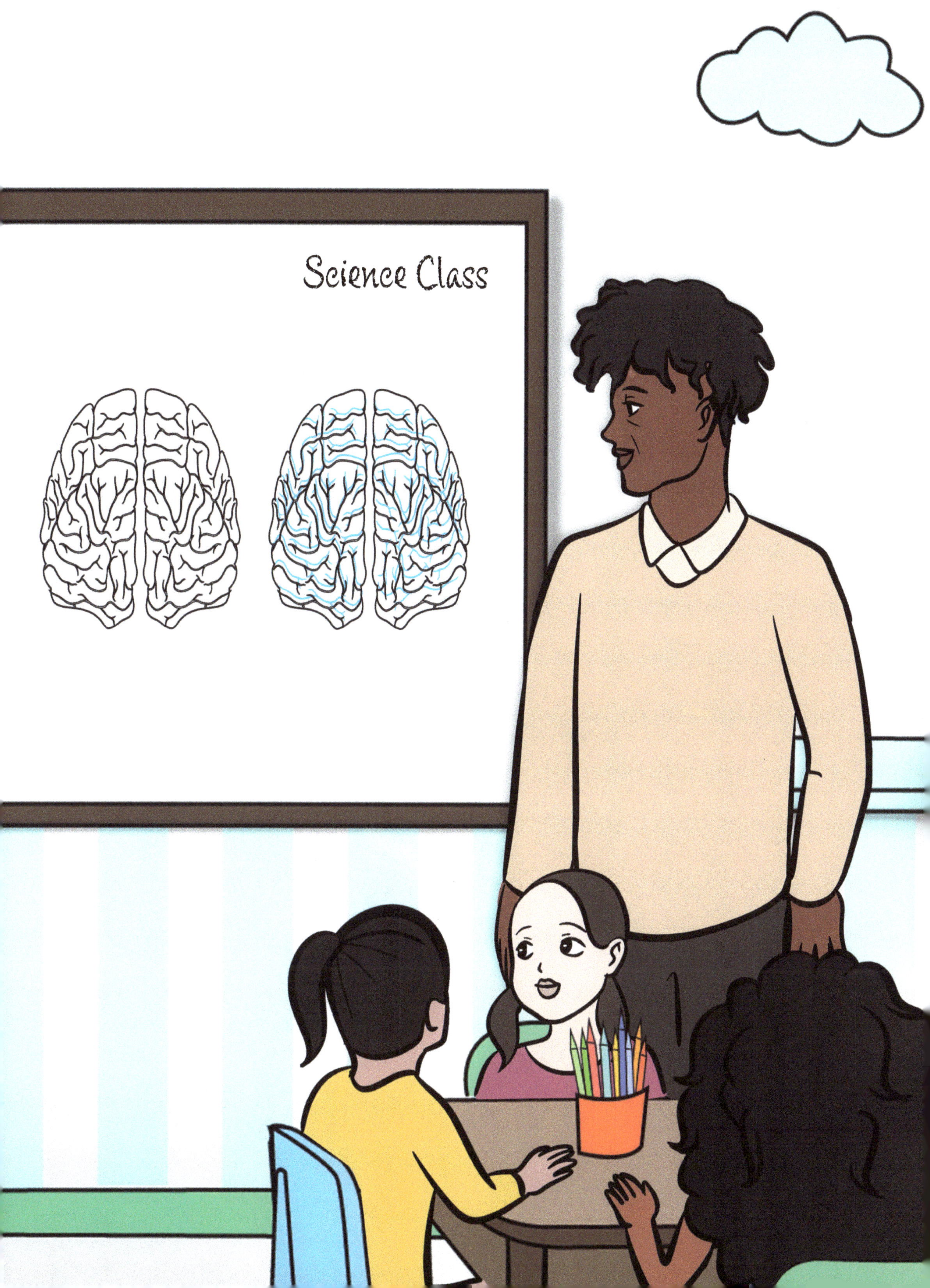

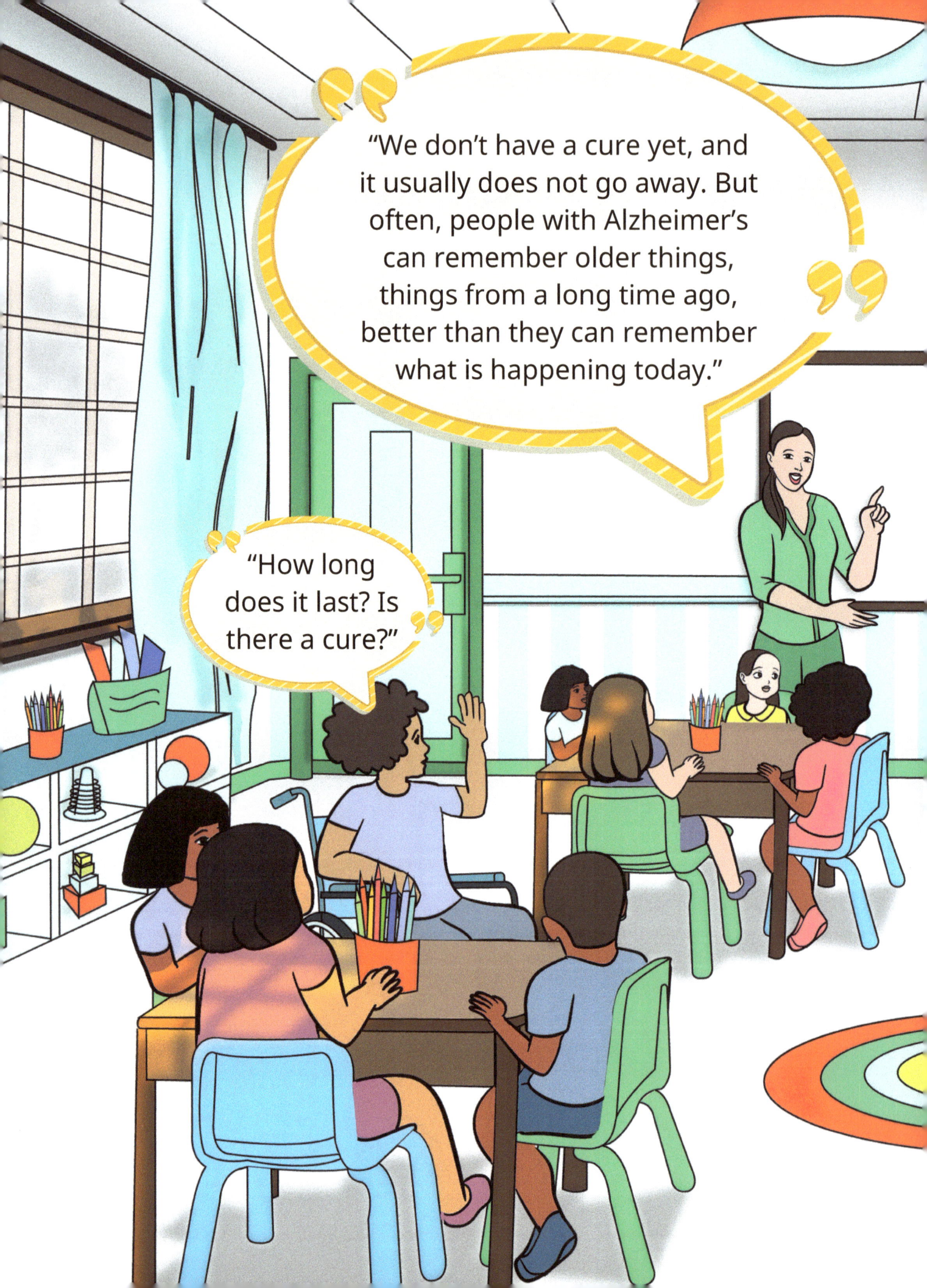

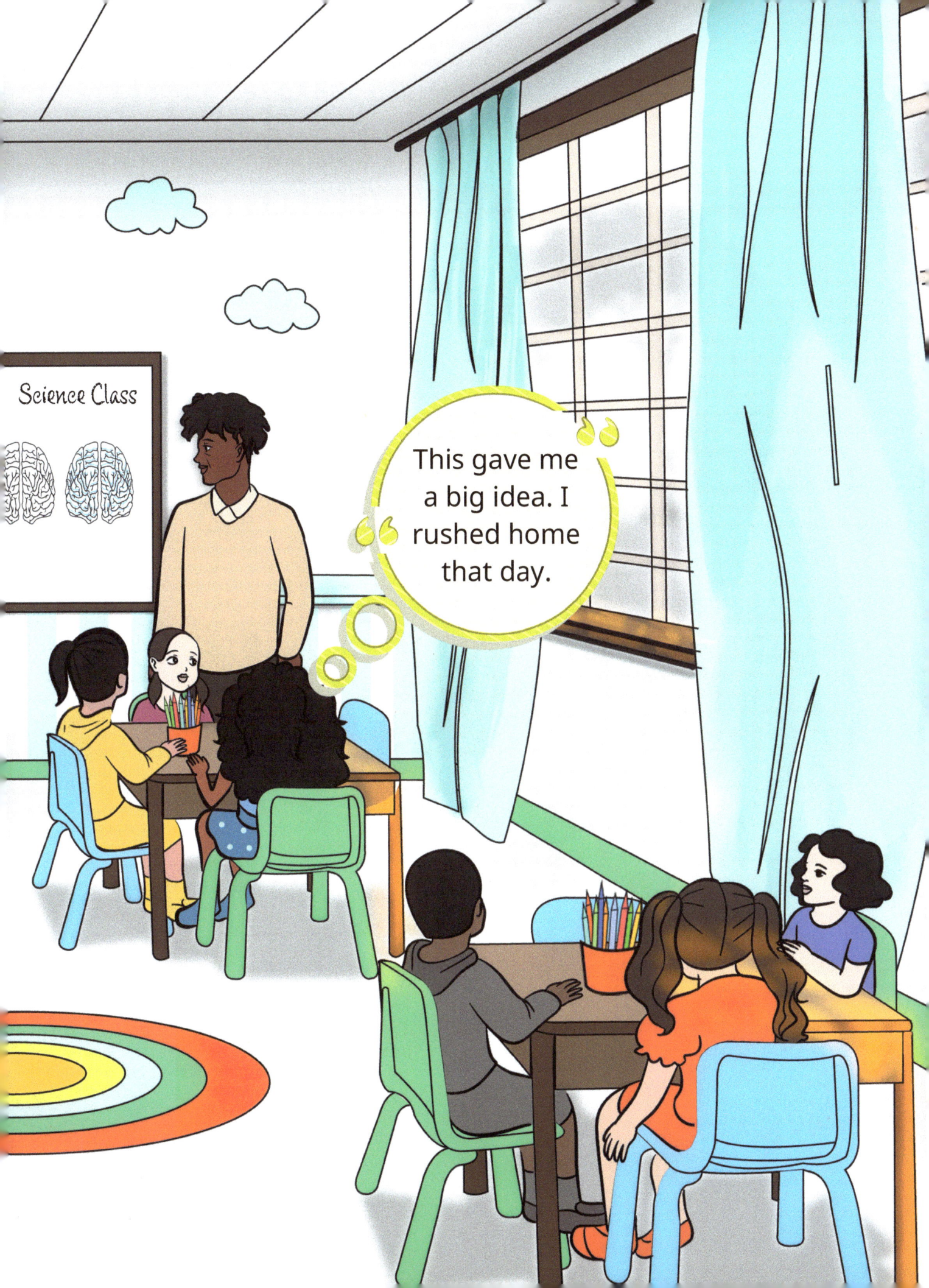

On our next visit to see Grandpa, he was the same, saying, "What is your name, little girl?" and "Who is that pretty lady with you?"
It was Grandma.

Grandpa didn't know my name.

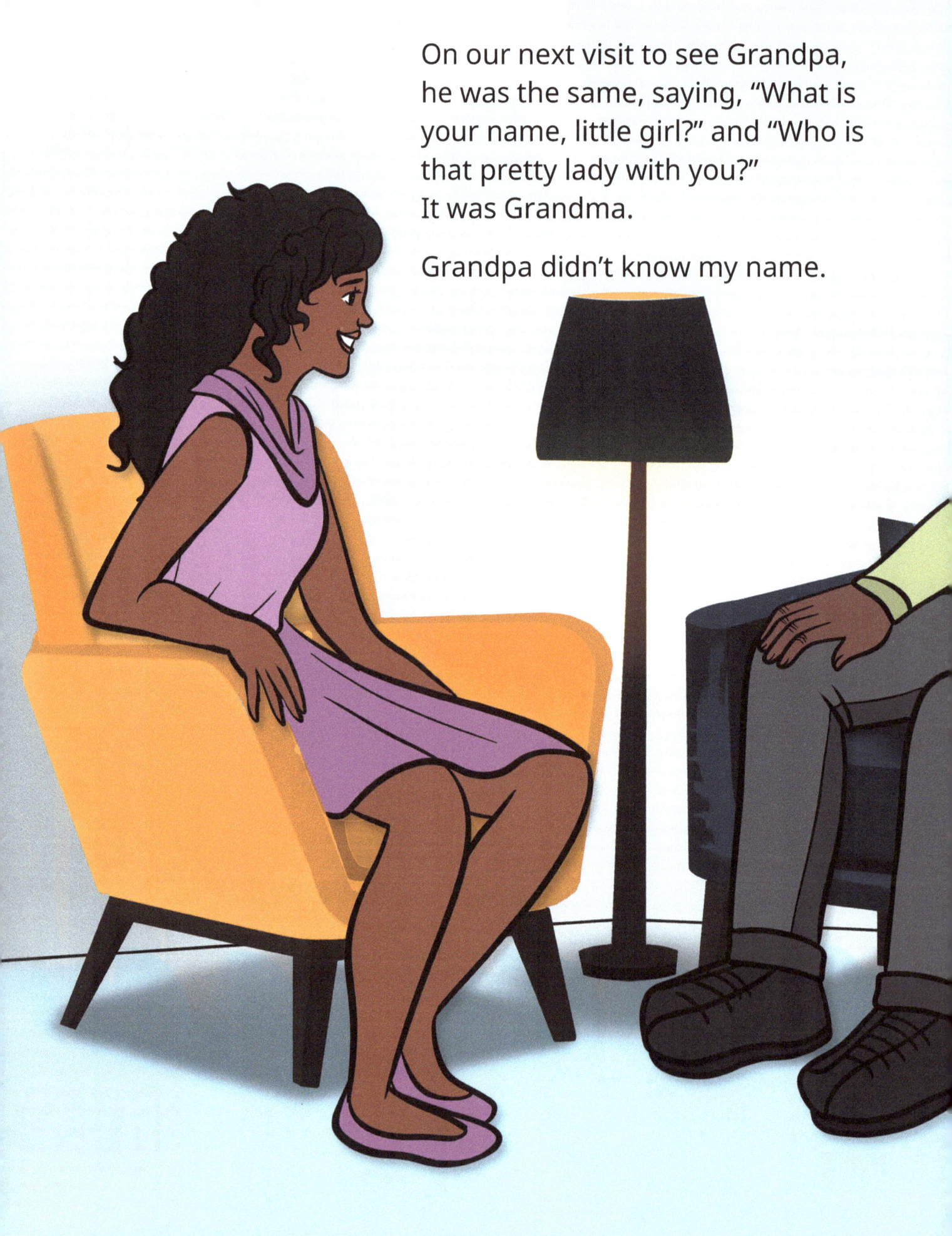

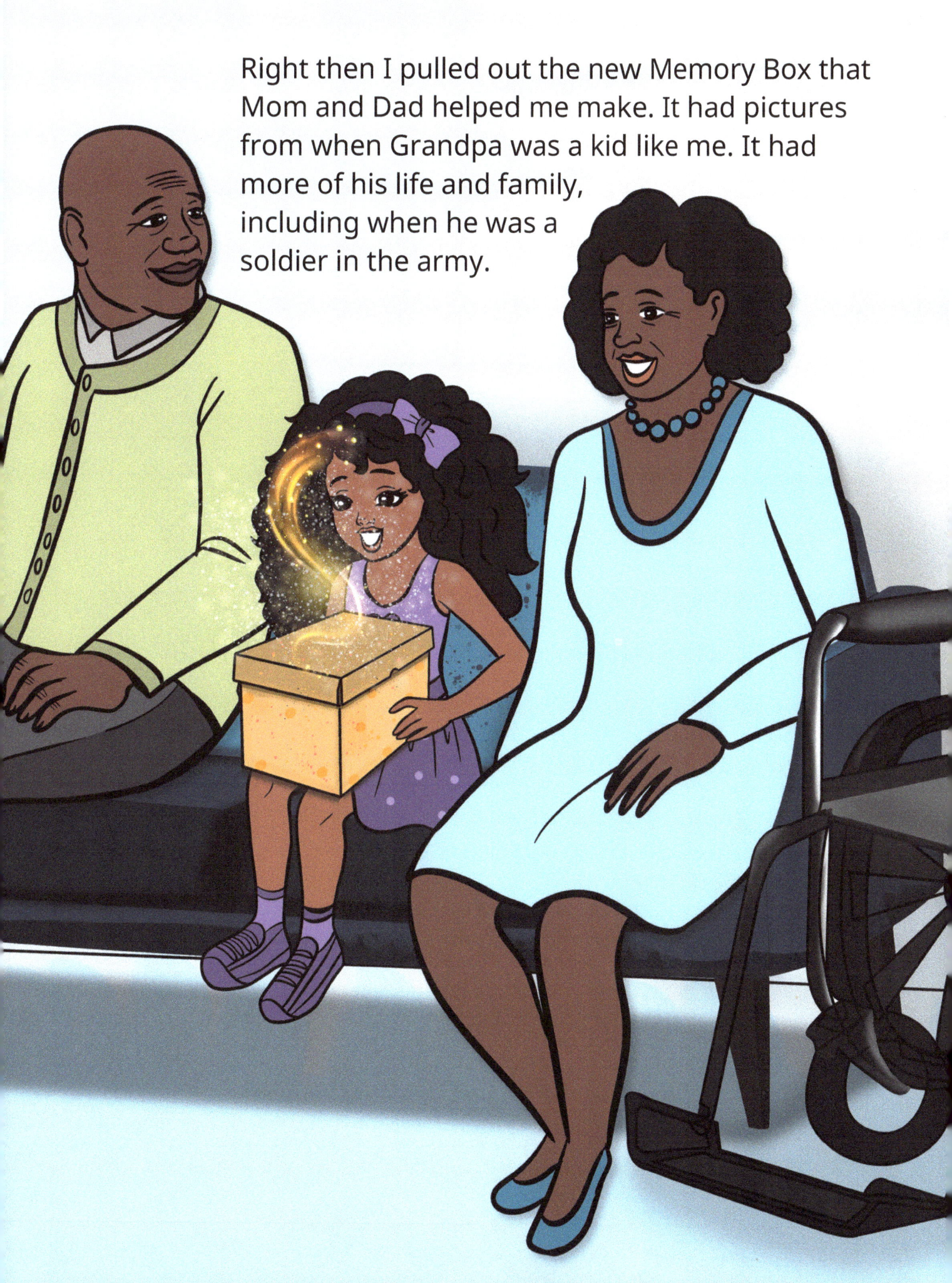

Right then I pulled out the new Memory Box that Mom and Dad helped me make. It had pictures from when Grandpa was a kid like me. It had more of his life and family, including when he was a soldier in the army.

We laughed a lot looking at all the pictures.

Pointing to a special picture of him and me, he explained, "And there—that is my little granddaughter."

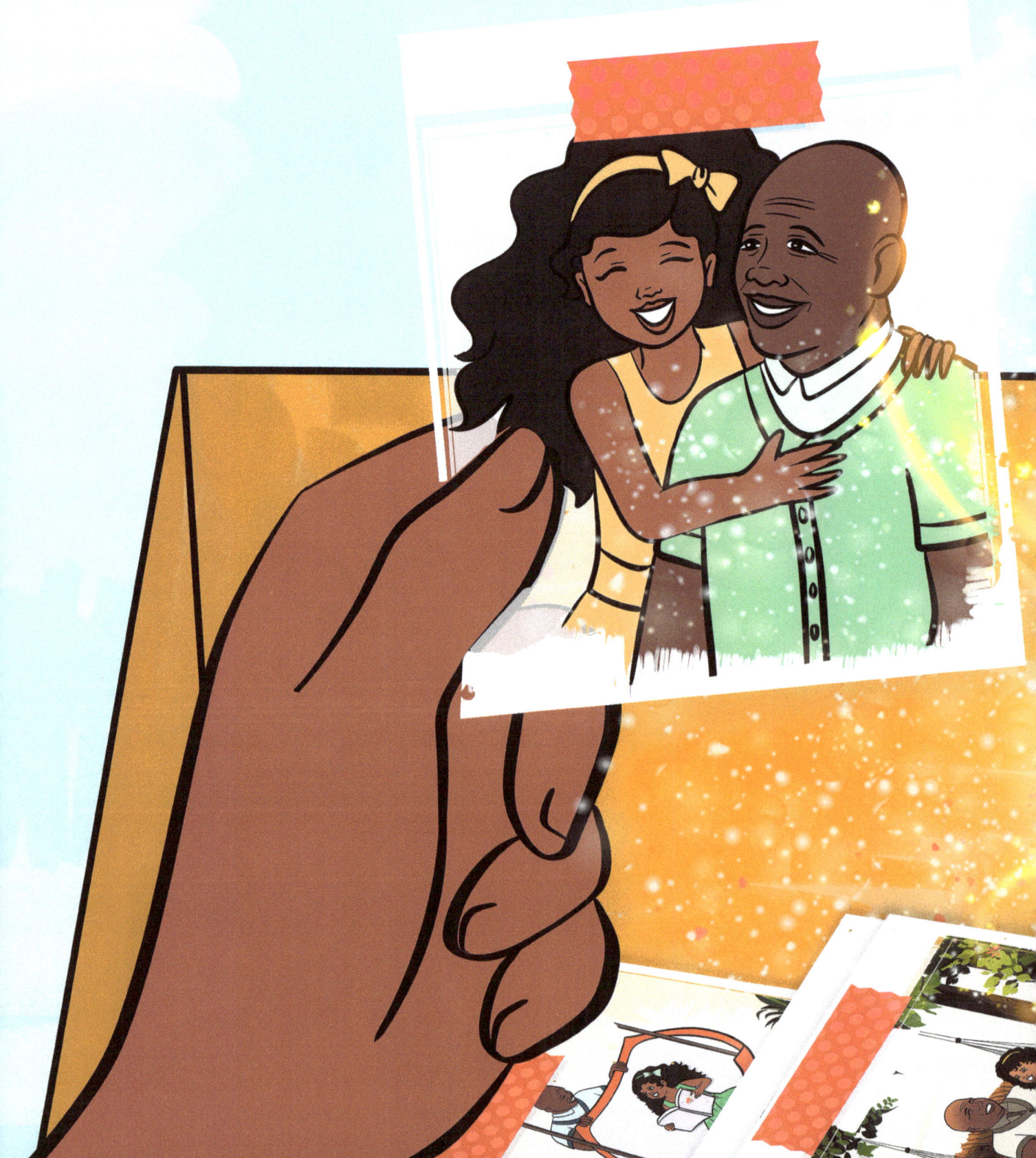

We prompted him, saying it was me, Charlotte. He nodded.

But I had a Big Surprise for Grandpa that day. I took his hand and started singing our favorite song.

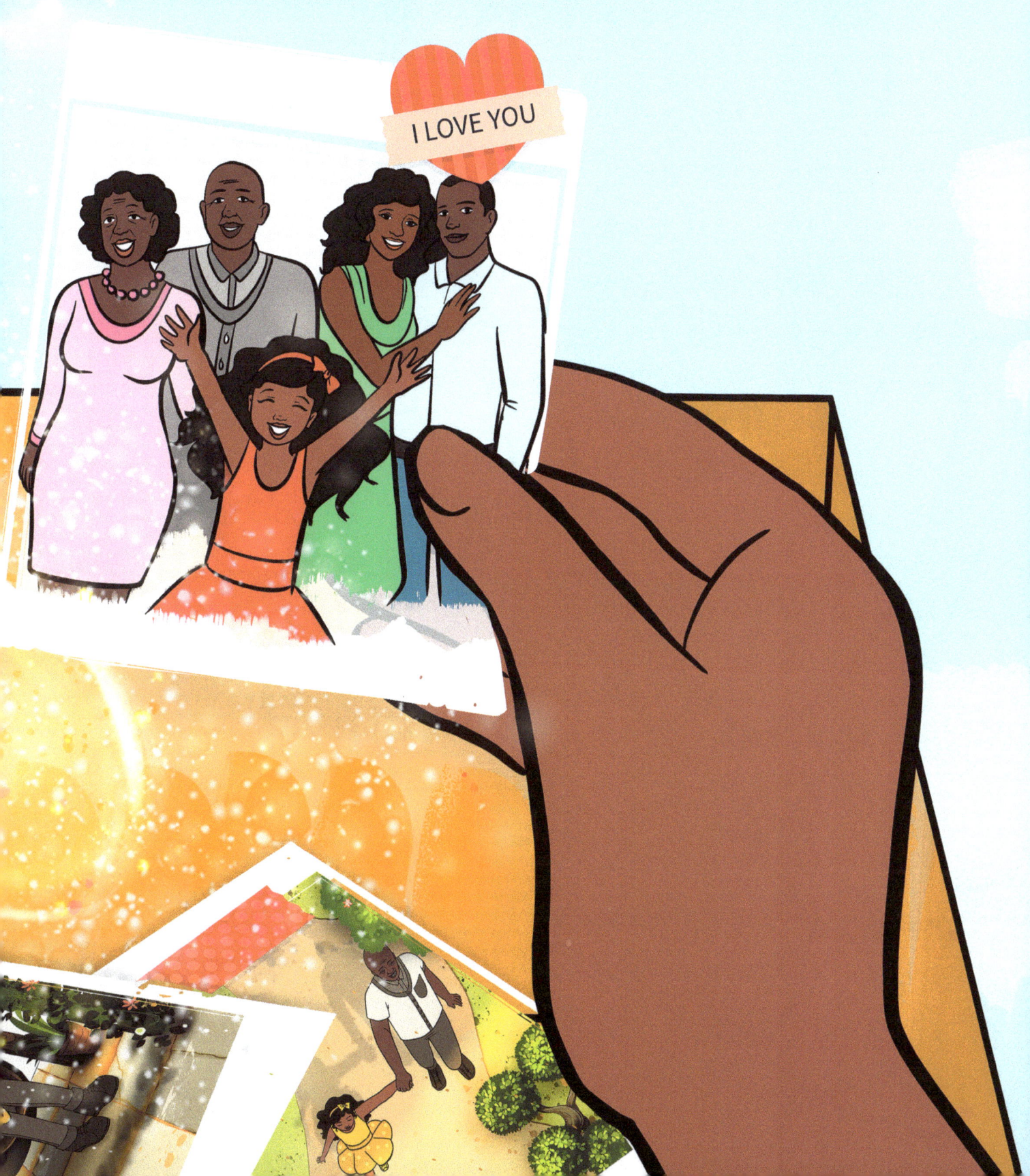

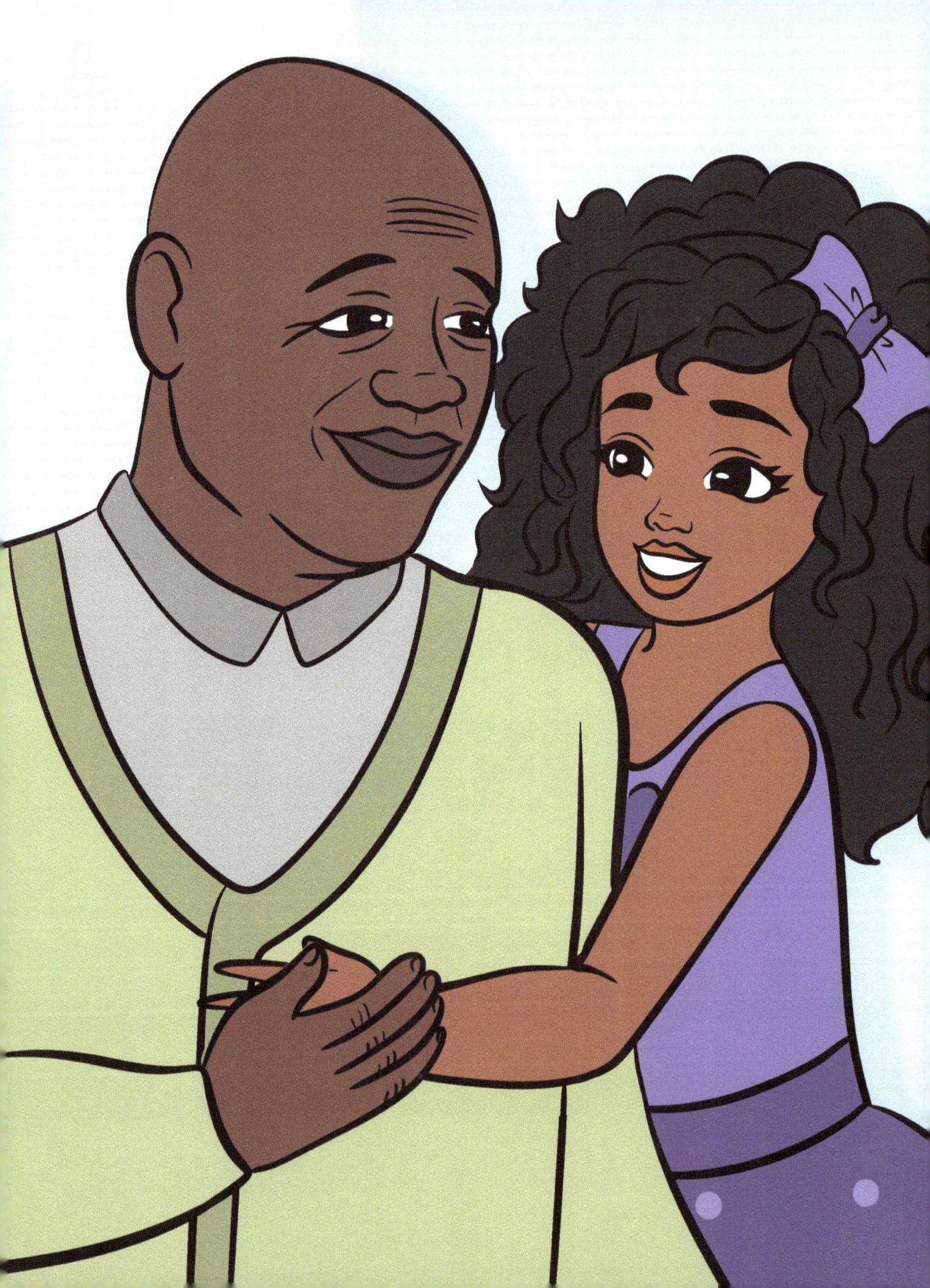

"Summertime and the livin' is easy. Fish are jumpin' and the cotton is high. Your daddy's rich and your ma is good lookin'. So hush, little baby, don't you cry.

"One of these mornings, you're gonna rise up singin'. You'll spread your wings, and you'll take to the sky. But till that mornin', there's nothin' can harm you. Yes, with Daddy and Mommy standin' by."

Grandpa smiled, then began to chuckle.

"How do you know my favorite song?"

I just gave him a big hug, and he hugged me right back. He looked into my eyes and said, "Charlotte."

The End

AUTHOR'S PERSPECTIVE

I am incredibly blessed to be part of bringing this story to life.

Why this book? I am a Professional Guardian. As a guardian, I manage the personal and fiduciary affairs of persons with Dementia, Alzheimer's Disease, and Developmental Disabilities. Also, my Uncle Jonah has Alzheimer's.

With my book, *Family and Professional Guardianship*, I aimed to help family guardians take care of their loved ones. As an extension of that, I became aware that each of these seniors had extended families, including many grandchildren.

How could I help them understand what was happening to Grandpa and Grandma? The answer: *The Memory Box*. I wanted to create a story that would help children understand this disease and celebrate the enduring power of love and family. I knew that I had to write this book for more than a year. It was like a constant itch that I couldn't get rid of. I thought, but who was I to write this book, and what made me think I could write a children's book?

Well, if you are reading this, then you know that you can never let self-doubt rule the day. One night, I woke up with an urge to write. It was 3:00 in the morning, and I thought to myself, *This can't be real; I never get up this early*. Despite this, I woke up three more times. On the third occasion, I got out of bed to write but laughed because I couldn't remember what I wanted to write. So, I went back to bed. However, the dream came to me again, and this time it was 5:00 AM.

This time, I immediately got out of bed, went into my study, which is really my guest bedroom, and began to write. The book poured out of me like running water. It was an experience like none I had ever had. I knew then that it was the hand of God. I no longer had thoughts about who may like the book or my ability to write it. I just trusted that if there was one child or family that could benefit from this inspired story, then it was worth it.

I'm deeply grateful to Zohra, the incredibly talented illustrator, who poured her heart and soul into these beautiful images. Her dedication and artistry have brought *The Memory Box & Charlotte's Big Surprise* to life in a way I could only have dreamed of.

To everyone who reads this book, thank you. I hope it brings comfort, understanding, and a renewed appreciation for the precious memories that connect us all.

It is my prayer that it will help your little ones understand that memories may fade, but love endures.

THE MEMORY BOX TEAM

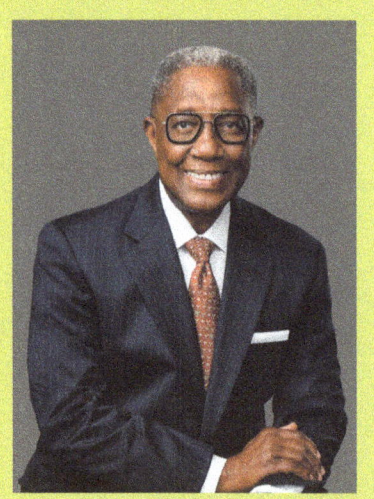

HOMER L. HARTAGE is the author of *Family and Professional Guardianship* and *The Memory Box*. These books expand on his work in Alzheimer's awareness, with *The Memory Box* focusing on young children and their love for elders with diminished memory.

Homer is the president of AgedCare, a professional guardianship company, and the Hartage Foundation, Inc., a Florida charity. As the oldest of six children raised by a single mother, he was a latch-key kid responsible for his two younger siblings. Caring for others comes naturally. He loves and cares deeply for people, especially those with the greatest needs

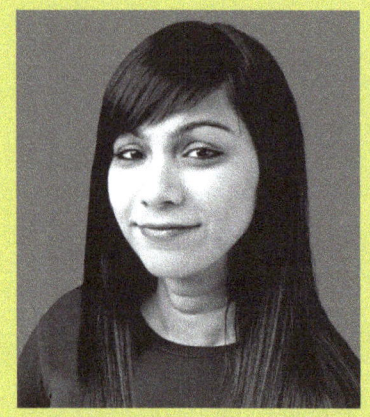

ZOHRA LAKHANI is a Harvard ALM graduate in Digital Media Design who connects with the universe through colors. As the VP of Communication & Creative Design for the Harvard Alumni Association of South Africa and a former Harvard Global Ambassador, she brings more than a decade of experience. Zohra has worked internationally in communication design, graphical illustration, digital media, branding, and advertising.

TRÚC ĐĂNG is an illustrator based in Hanoi, Vietnam, with more than six years of experience in the field. She has worked on numerous projects, including book illustrations, editorial pieces, and visual storytelling for a variety of clients. Trúc's work is known for its thoughtful details, expressive characters, and vibrant use of color, often inspired by her love for nature, culture, and everyday life.

Special thanks to my editor, E. Lee Caleca. I have turned to her over and over for her keen insight, dedication to improving the copy, and bringing the story to an impactful conclusion.

Special thanks to my dedicated staff at AgedCare, you help so many with your dedication to caring and service to others. www.agedcareguardian.com

In Loving Memory of Frieda Schachner, A.B., my beloved chemistry teacher at Snyder High School, Jersey City, NJ, you instilled so much knowledge, passion, and inspiration in all of us. Your influence continues to shape our lives, and your legacy will always be cherished.